Prostate
Problems

Jane Smith BSc (Hons)
Medical Editor and Writer, Bristol

&

David Gillatt ChM, FRCS
Consultant Urologist,
Bristol Urological Institute, Southmead Hospital, Bristol

ILLUSTRATIONS BY ALEXANDER JAMES

Headway · Hodder & Stoughton

Other titles published in this series

Breast Lumps
Hernias
Hysterectomy & alternative operations
Varicose Veins
Male and Female Sterilisation
Cataracts
Skin Cancers

A catalogue record of this publication is available from the British Library.

ISBN 0 340 679077

First published 1996
Impression number   10   9   8   7   6   5   4   3   2   1
Year   1999   1998   1997   1996

Copyright © 1996 Jane Smith

Typeset by Wearset, Boldon, Tyne and Wear.
Printed in Great Britain for Hodder & Stoughton Educational, a division of
Hodder Headline Plc, 338 Euston Road, London NW1 3BH by Cox & Wyman Ltd,
Reading, Berks.

Cover: detail from 'The Creation of Adam' by Michelangelo, Sistine Chapel,
Bridgeman Art Library, London.

Contents

General preface to the series

Two people having the same operation can have quite different experiences, but one feeling that is common to many is that things might have been easier if they had had a better idea of what to expect. Some people are reluctant to ask questions, and many forget what they are told, sometimes because they are anxious, and sometimes because they do not really understand the explanations they are given.

In most medical centres in Britain today, the emphasis is more on patient involvement than at any time in the past. It is now generally accepted that it is important for people to understand what their treatment entails, both in terms of reducing their stress and thus aiding their recovery, and of making their care more straightforward for the medical staff involved.

The books in this series have been written with the aim of giving people comprehensive information about each of the medical conditions covered, about the treatment they are likely to be offered, and about what may happen during their post-operative recovery period. Armed with this knowledge, you should have the confidence to question, and to take part in the decisions made.

Going in to hospital for the first time can be a daunting experience, and therefore the books describe the procedures involved, and identify and explain the roles of the hospital staff with whom you are likely to come into contact.

Anaesthesia is explained in general terms, and the options available for a particular operation are described in each book.

There may be complications following any operation – usually minor but none the less worrying for the person involved – and the common ones are described and explained. Now that less time is spent in hospital following most non-emergency operations, knowing what to expect in the days following surgery, and what to do if a complication does arise, is more important than ever before.

Where relevant, the books include a section of exercises and advice to help you to get back to normal and to deal with the everyday activities which can be difficult or painful in the first few days after an operation.

Doctors and nurses, like members of any profession, use a jargon, and they often forget that many of the terms that are familiar to them are not part of everyday language for most of us. Care has been taken to make the books easily understandable by everyone, and each book has a list of simple explanations of the medical terms you may come across.

Most doctors and nurses are more than willing to explain and to discuss problems with patients, but they often assume that if you do not ask questions, you either do not want to know or you know already. Questions and answers are given in every book to help you to draw up your own list to take with you when you see your family doctor or consultant.

Each book also has a section of case histories of people who have experienced the particular operation themselves. These are included to give you an idea of the problems which can arise, problems which may sometimes seem relatively trivial to others but which can be distressing to those directly concerned.

Although the majority of people are satisfied with the medical care they receive, things can go wrong. If you do feel you need to make a complaint about something that happened, or did not happen, during your treatment, each book has a section which deals in detail with how to go about this.

It was the intention in writing these books to help to take

some of the worry out of having an operation. It is not knowing what to expect, and the feeling of being involved in some process over which we have no control, and which we do not fully understand, that makes us anxious. The books in the series *Your Operation* should help to remove some of that anxiety and make you feel less like a car being serviced, and more like part of the team of people who are working together to cure your medical problem and put you back on the road to health.

You may not know *all* there is to know about a particular condition when you have read the book related to it, but you will know more than enough to prepare yourself for your operation. You may decide you do not want to go ahead with surgery. Although this is not the authors' intention, they will be happy that you have been given enough information to feel confident to make your own decision, and to take an active part in your own care. After all, it is *your* operation.

Jane Smith
Bristol, 1996

Preface

One in three men over the age of 50 has difficulty passing urine, in most cases caused by an enlarged prostate gland pressing on the urethra which carries urine from the bladder. The prostate gland begins to grow during a man's thirties, but is usually not significantly enlarged until middle age or later. It may remain symptomless or it may give rise to urinary symptoms of varying degree.

Apart from enlargement of the prostate (known as benign prostatic hyperplasia), urinary problems can also be caused by inflammation or infection of the prostate (prostatitis) and by prostate cancer. Again, prostate cancer in its early stages may not cause any symptoms and there is currently discussion in Britain as to the potential benefits of introducing nationwide screening programmes to detect the presence of cancer before it has had a chance to spread, when treatment is less effective.

Treatment for prostate problems may involve regular monitoring, the use of drugs or surgery and, in some cases of prostate cancer, hormone therapy or radiotherapy. In the UK each year, some 45 000 men have prostate operations and approximately 14 000 new cases of prostate cancer are diagnosed.

The aim of this book is to provide clear explanations of the three main causes of prostate problems, their symptoms, the investigations done to enable a diagnosis to be made, the treatment options, both medical and surgical, and the possible side-effects of surgery.

Many men are likely to experience some degree of prostate-related symptoms as they get older, and the information contained in this book should help them to understand the causes and to be fully aware of what is involved in any proposed treatment. It is hoped also that the book will be useful to the wives and other family members of men with prostate problems, whose anxieties may sometimes be overlooked and whose questions may remain unanswered.

Jane Smith
David Gillatt
1996

Acknowledgements

We are particularly grateful to Mr Martin Lancashire, Consultant in Urology at the Alexandra Hospital, Redditch; to Dr John Graham, Consultant in Clinical Oncology at the Bristol Oncology Centre; and to Heather Gould, Clinical Research Nurse in Urology at Southmead Hospital, Bristol.

Thanks are also due to the men who related their own experiences of prostate problems for the section on case histories.

CHAPTER 1

Introduction

The prostate is a gland which is present in men and situated at the base of the bladder. It encircles the urethra through which urine is transported from the bladder and down the penis. Because of its proximity to the urethra, problems which affect the prostate lead to problems in passing urine.

There are three main causes of prostate problems which will be dealt with in this book. Enlargement of the prostate due to **benign prostatic hyperplasia (BPH)** occurs naturally with age and tends to cause urinary symptoms of greater or lesser degree. The prostate gland can also be affected by an inflammatory condition called **prostatitis**, and by **prostate cancer**. Before discussing these conditions in detail, it is useful to have some understanding of the structure and function of the prostate gland and of some of the other male reproductive organs.

THE MALE REPRODUCTIVE ORGANS

The **urethra** in both men and women transports urine from the bladder. In men it also carries the **semen** which is ejaculated following sexual arousal. The male urethra is about 20 cm (8 inches) long and extends from the neck of the bladder to the bulbous tip of the penis.

In the male fetus, two **testes** (or **testicles**) develop near the kidneys, but by birth they have normally descended through a canal in the abdominal wall and into the **scrotum**. Each testis is an oval, glandular organ, about 4 cm (1.5 inches) long by 2.5 cm (1 inch) wide. Sperm are produced within **seminiferous tubules** in the testes and pass via a system of ducts and tubes to be

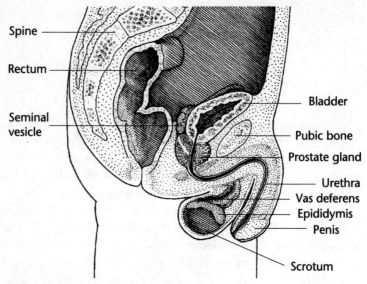

Spine

Rectum

Seminal vesicle

Bladder

Pubic bone

Prostate gland

Urethra

Vas deferens

Epididymis

Penis

Scrotum

The male reproductive organs.

stored in the two **seminal vesicles** which lie at the base of the bladder adjacent to the prostate gland. When ejaculation occurs, large numbers of sperm, together with secretions from the prostate, are discharged into the urethra as semen. Muscles in the neck of the bladder contract during ejaculation, closing the bladder off and preventing semen passing back into it.

The prostate gland

The prostate gland is about the size and shape of a walnut and is partially enclosed in a capsule of muscle and connective tissue. Its surface is covered with a rich supply of blood vessels and nerves, and it is divided into a left and right lobe by a longitudinal furrow. The prostate secretes a milky fluid into the semen which is thought to contribute to the fertility of sperm, although its precise function is not fully understood.

2

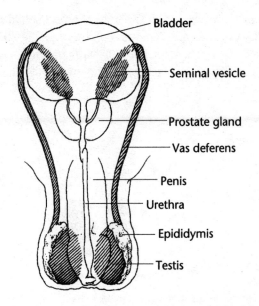

The male genital tract. This is a schematic representation; the bladder as shown here is empty and will expand when full of urine.

The growth and function of the prostate gland are regulated by the complex interaction of numerous steroid and other hormones, primarily by the male sex hormone **testosterone** which is produced by the testes. With age, the hormonal regulation tends to break down and the prostate gland enlarges. Its growth can result in symptoms varying in severity from an increased need to urinate to total urine retention for which immediate treatment is necessary.

BENIGN PROSTATIC HYPERPLASIA

The condition causes benign enlargement of the prostate and is most common in men over the age of 50, although growth of (and microscopic changes in) the prostate gland may begin in their thirties and there is a phase of accelerated growth around 40. Benign prostatic hyperplasia is present in about 50 per cent of men by the age of 60 and in about 80 per cent in their eighties.

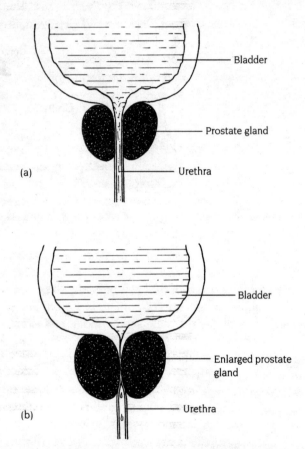

(a)

Bladder

Prostate gland

Urethra

(b)

Bladder

Enlarged prostate gland

Urethra

Enlargement of the prostate gland. (a) A normal prostate allows urine to flow through the urethra. (b) As the prostate enlarges, it constricts the urethra and blocks the passage of urine from the bladder.

Symptoms

As the prostate gland grows, it may constrict the urethra, causing a variety of urinary symptoms. Although symptoms arise if the urethra becomes blocked, the degree of obstruction is not necessarily directly related to the size of the prostate: it may be partially dependent on the tone of the prostatic muscles.

The syndrome caused by benign prostatic hyperplasia is often called **prostatism**. It involves symptoms of urinary obstruction, such as decreased or hesitant urine flow and a feeling of incomplete emptying of the bladder (see p.14). Symptoms of irritation may also occur if the bladder muscles have to work harder to overcome the obstruction. Irritative symptoms include a sudden urge to urinate and a need to urinate frequently during the night, although similar symptoms may occur with various other conditions. In a small number of cases, complications can develop such as acute or chronic urinary retention (see p.10).

Although benign prostatic hyperplasia is a progressive condition, its symptoms do not necessarily worsen. Left untreated, it can sometimes have the following effects.

* *Hypertrophy of the bladder*: thickening of the muscles of the bladder wall, which in itself is not serious.
* *Urinary stasis*: the retention of a volume of urine in the bladder after urination (micturition). As the bladder is normally kept clean by emptying, bacteria can become established in any urine retained, leading to *urinary tract infections*. Infection can be recurrent and may result in cystitis.
* *Hydronephrosis*: enlargement of the drainage system of the kidneys due to the accumulation of urine, sometimes as a result of urinary retention. This can occasionally lead to kidney damage or failure.

* *Detrusor instability*: overactivity of the muscular layers of the bladder wall, leading to irritative symptoms.
* *Detrusor decompensation*: inability of the muscles of the bladder to contract properly, causing the bladder to become atonic (see Atonic bladder, p.11) and resulting in chronic urinary retention.

Causes

The causes of benign prostatic hyperplasia are not fully understood, but it is known that ageing and the testicular hormones produced by functioning testes are essential factors in its development.

PROSTATITIS

There are three forms of prostatitis, all of which tend to occur in relatively young men, commonly between the ages of 20 and 50. Although prostatitis does not involve enlargement of the prostate gland, the symptoms may be similar. Diagnosis is broadly clinical, although a transrectal ultrasound scan (see p.21) may also be useful.

Bacterial prostatitis

Bacterial prostatitis can be acute, with symptoms similar to those of urine infection: pain when passing urine, bladder pain, fever and frequent micturition. There is also a chronic form of the infection, the symptoms of which are sometimes brought on by bowel motions and tend to recur. They may include back pain, discomfort around the lower abdomen and genitals, and pain when passing urine. Bacteria can be grown from a urine specimen and identified in a laboratory so that the appropriate antibiotic can be selected for treatment.

Abacterial prostatitis

Abacterial prostatitis has symptoms similar to the bacterial form but which tend to come and go and can be fairly vague. They include discomfort around the genitals, between the scrotum and anus (the area known as the **perineum**), in the lower abdomen and low back. However, no bacteria are apparent in the urine or prostatic fluid. A long course of antibiotic treatment may be successful, although a chronic condition can be difficult to clear up completely.

Prostadynia

Prostadynia means prostate pain and this type of prostatitis is accompanied by discomfort in the prostatic region. Its cause is difficult to identify and treatment of its symptoms is often the best that can be done.

PROSTATE CANCER

Prostate cancer is rare before the age of 50. Over 95 per cent of prostate cancers are **adenocarcinomas**, a type of **carcinoma** which is usually slow growing. (A carcinoma is a cancer of epithelial tissue which lines structures such as the prostate and bladder.)

What is a cancer?

Normally, cells have a finite lifespan, after which they die and are replaced, but sometimes the control mechanisms break down, resulting in abnormal growth of the tissue – a swelling known as a **tumour**. Tumours can be **benign** (non-cancerous) or **malignant** (a cancer). Although benign tumours can cause pain and interfere with the normal function of adjacent organs as they enlarge, they are rarely life-threatening and usually respond to treatment. They do not spread to other parts of the body, remaining localised at their site of development. Malignant tumours, on the other hand, destroy nearby cells as they grow and can eventually spread via the blood or lymphatic system to other parts of the body, where they form secondary tumours known as **metastases**. The lymphatic vessels transport lymph, a clear fluid which drains waste away from the tissues. As the lymph passes through glands (known as **lymph nodes**) at various sites around the body, unwanted substances such as cancer cells are filtered out. Spread of a cancer is therefore often to the regional lymph nodes in the first instance. The process of spread is known as **metastasis**.

Symptoms

A small prostate tumour may be symptomless and may even remain undetected during rectal examination (see p.18). As it grows, the first symptom may be difficulty urinating, although this is more commonly a symptom of benign prostatic hyperplasia.

Prostate cancer tends to spread to the lymph nodes and bones, especially those of the hip and lower back. Bone pain is therefore often a symptom of spread of the disease. The various stages in the development of prostate cancer can be determined by testing. Treatment at an early stage, before spread has occurred, is most likely to be effective.

Causes

The causes of prostate cancer are not fully understood, but it is known that its growth is stimulated by the hormone testosterone. There appears to be a genetic link with the disease, which occurs more commonly in Negro races and is very uncommon in people of oriental origin. However, the incidence of prostate cancer increases in Orientals (particularly the Japanese) who move from their country of origin to America, although it still remains lower than that of Caucasians or Negroes. This fact indicates an additional environmental link, possibly diet.

The possibility of a genetic association is further supported by the fact that the risk of getting prostate cancer is at least twice as great as normal for a man with a first-degree relative (father, brother or uncle) who developed the disease before the age of 65.

Various other predisposing factors have been implicated, such as working in a nuclear power station or coming into contact with selenium, a constituent of some fertilisers used by farmers. However, there is less evidence to support suggestions that other factors, such as having a vasectomy, increase the risk of developing prostate cancer.

Screening for prostate cancer

There is currently controversy surrounding the potential advantages which could be gained from introducing screening for prostate cancer in the UK. In the USA, all men over the age of 45 are advised to be screened, and the programme there has led to 200 000 new cases of prostate cancer being diagnosed each year, and an increase in radical surgery. However, there are as yet no plans to set up mass screening programmes in the UK, although there is a call for clinical trials to assess the effects they could have. It is predicted that, within the next few years, prostate cancer will become the most commonly diagnosed malignancy in men.

The supporters of screening point out that in its early stages prostate cancer is often symptomless, and that in about half of the 14 000 new cases diagnosed in the UK each year, spread to the bones has already occurred. Most prostate cancers are first detected during investigations of urinary problems. However, treatment at an early stage of development is most likely to be effective, and routine screening could therefore have a significant effect on mortality.

Those who do not support nationwide screening feel that the vast majority of men with prostate cancer but no symptoms would gain no benefit from treatment as the disease can remain latent for years in elderly men and most are likely to die from other causes. They therefore consider that screening would cause unnecessary anxiety and that the possible side-effects of treatment, including impotence and incontinence, would not be justified.

Small-scale screening trials have already been run in some parts of the UK. For example, during a recent trial involving 5000 men, 65 were found to have prostate cancer, although all were symptomless, and a further 45 had pre-cancerous changes in their prostate tissue. The debate continues.

OTHER CAUSES OF URINARY PROBLEMS

Some of the conditions described below can be associated with prostate disease, although all may have other causes.

Urinary retention

Apart from sometimes being caused by prostate problems, urinary retention can also be precipitated by, for example, a prolapsed disc, a hip operation, constipation or a blockage elsewhere in the urethra.

Acute urinary retention may develop suddenly and be accompanied by pain. It can be precipitated in the early stages of a prostate condition by constipation or by voluntarily retaining urine, for example when you need to urinate but are unable to get to a toilet. The initial treatment is to insert a catheter (see p.16), either through the penis or suprapubically. If there is a precipitating cause other than enlargement of the prostate, the catheter can be removed, once the cause has been treated, to see if urine can be passed spontaneously. When acute urinary retention is associated with benign prostate enlargement, an operation is usually necessary to reduce the size of the prostate gland before urine can be passed voluntarily.

Chronic urinary retention occurs when the bladder is unable to empty completely over a prolonged period of time. It does not cause pain and may be accompanied by symptoms such as dribbling of urine after urination, known as **overflow incontinence**. Your abdomen may distend as your bladder enlarges, and you may notice your waistband becoming tighter. If the situation continues for some time and the kidneys are unable to drain into the bladder, kidney failure may be the first apparent sign that something is wrong. Kidney failure in its early stages is usually symptomless, but as it progresses you may feel generally unwell and sick and may begin to lose weight.

Treatment of chronic urinary retention may involve a period of catheterisation to try to improve kidney function. If the prostate gland is enlarged, surgery may be necessary before the catheter can be removed.

Atonic bladder

The symptoms of an atonic bladder may be similar to those of chronic urinary retention, namely a full bladder, difficulty passing urine and possibly incontinence. The condition occurs when the bladder fails to empty properly and, as it fills up, the muscles of its wall lose their tone, i.e. their ability to contract and squeeze out the urine efficiently. The bladder will eventually become like a floppy sac.

Surgery to reduce the size of an enlarged prostate may fail to improve an atonic bladder and, for older men with mild symptoms, treatment is often unnecessary. However, if infection develops because there is a stagnant pool of urine left in the bladder, catheterisation may be required, sometimes permanently.

Irritable bladder

If the bladder muscle becomes overactive, it may cause urinary symptoms such as the more frequent passage of small amounts of urine and increased urgency, which sometimes results in the leakage of urine before a toilet can be reached. Similar symptoms can also be due to irritation of the bladder by infection, stones or tumours. An irritable bladder with no underlying cause can be treated with anticholinergic drugs, given as tablets, to act on the nerves to the bladder (see p.27). However, if the bladder muscles have become overactive as a result of an enlarged prostate gland causing urinary obstruction, anticholinergic drugs can make the condition worse.

Urethral stricture

Narrowing of the urethra may have no obvious cause. In the past is was commonly the result of physical damage, for example following an accident, or of infection such as gonorrhoea. It is now more likely to develop after surgery, including transurethral resection of the prostate (see p.28), or after catheterisation. Its symptoms include a reduction in the urinary stream, and less powerful, more frequent urination.

Nocturnal polyuria

Normally, antidiuretic hormone, which is produced by the brain, acts to reduce the function of the kidneys at night so that they produce less urine. However, as your 'body clock' alters with age, you may find that you pass large amounts of urine during the night, possibly as much as you do during daytime. This condition is known as nocturnal polyuria.

It may be helpful to reduce your fluid intake in the evenings, but there are drugs available which might be more effective. A diuretic tablet such as frusemide can be taken in the early evening to make you pass a lot of urine before you go to bed, thus reducing the amount you produce during the night. Alternatively, you may be prescribed desmopressin, a synthetic form of antidiuretic hormone which is given as a nasal spray or tablets. If taken just before you go to bed, desmopressin may be successful in turning your kidneys off for the night. However, as it can cause fluid retention in people with other medical problems, its use is not always appropriate.

CHAPTER 2

Investigations and decisions

If you have troublesome urinary symptoms, tests may be done to discover their cause before any decision is made about treatment.

SYMPTOMS AND SIGNS

[**Symptoms** are what the patient complains of, for example pain. **Signs** are what the doctor looks for, such as a swelling.]

Prostate enlargement or disease can be present without any symptoms and there can be various other causes of urinary problems, such as kidney or bladder infections or stones. However, when the symptoms described below occur in men over the age of 50, they are often due to disease or enlargement of the prostate gland and you should consult your family doctor if you experience persistent and troublesome problems.

* *Hesitancy*: having to wait to pass urine, the flow of which may be slow and/or interrupted and little improved by straining.
* *Urgency*: a sudden and possibly frequent need to urinate.
* *Frequency*: urinating more often than previously.
* *Urge incontinence*: a sudden need to urinate which may result in urine leaking before you reach the toilet.
* *Nocturia*: being woken during the night by the need to urinate, although often only very small amounts of urine are actually passed. (This symptom is distinct from nocturnal

polyuria (see p.12) which involves passing large amounts of urine during the night.)

Medical advice should always be sought for any other signs and symptoms such as blood in your urine (which is occasionally related to prostate problems) or an inability to urinate despite the urge to do so (which may be due to urine retention).

VISITING YOUR FAMILY DOCTOR

Whether through reluctance to undergo tests and examination, a fear of what may be discovered, or an optimistic belief that the problems will go away, many men put off visiting their doctor for

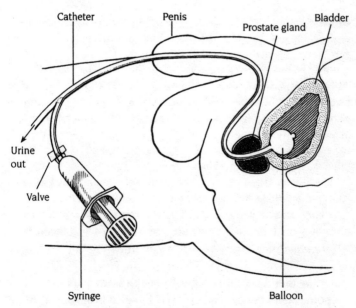

A urinary catheter. The catheter is held in place in the bladder by a balloon which is inflated using a water-filled syringe.

some time after urinary symptoms first become apparent. However, it is important to seek medical advice if troublesome problems persist, and helpful to be able to give your doctor a note of when and how often you have been urinating and of any other relevant details.

If your symptoms are not severe, your doctor may decide to monitor the situation for a while and you may be asked to return for another appointment some weeks later or if your problems worsen. Alternatively, your doctor may prescribe a course of drugs or refer you to a consultant or to a hospital out-patient clinic for tests.

If you develop painful, acute urine retention, you will require immediate treatment, and your doctor may insert a catheter through your penis to drain the urine from your bladder.

Urinary catheters The treatment for some urinary symptoms involves the insertion of a catheter to drain urine from the bladder. A catheter is a narrow, flexible tube which is coated with local anaesthetic before being carefully inserted into the bladder, either into the penis and through the urethra or through a small incision made in the lower abdominal wall. (The latter is known as a **suprapubic** catheter.) A small balloon at the tip of the catheter is then inflated with fluid to hold it in place in the bladder. After insertion, the other end of the catheter is attached to a bag into which the urine drains and which may be taped to your leg.

The catheter is removed by withdrawing the fluid from the balloon into a syringe attached to the lower end of the tube and gently sliding it out of the penis. The procedure may cause some discomfort. A suprapubic catheter is removed in much the same way, and a pressure dressing is then placed over the small wound.

You may then be sent straight to hospital for examination or an appointment may be made for you to see a **urologist** within a few days. (A urologist is a doctor who specialises in the urinary system and the diseases which affect it.) If it is necessary for the catheter to remain in place for any length of time, the small bag attached to it will probably be taped to your leg and you will be shown how to empty it as it fills with urine. You will also be given a larger bag to attach to the small one for night-time drainage.

EXAMINATIONS AND TESTS

If you require examination or treatment, you may be referred to a urology clinic (or possibly a **flow clinic**) at a hospital. Before your appointment, you may be sent a chart on which to record how often you need to urinate and the volume of urine you pass over a period of several days. Take the completed chart with you to your clinic appointment. Tests will be done at the clinic to assess the cause of your symptoms and the severity of any bladder obstruction. A decision will then be made about whether treatment is necessary and, if so, what type of treatment is appropriate.

Day	Day-time Time/volume (ml)			Night-time Time/volume (ml)	
1	7:30 am 200	11 am couldn't measure	3:30 pm 300	2 am 200	6 am awoke wet
	6 pm 300	11 pm 400			
2					

A typical frequency/outflow chart. You may be asked to keep a record of your urine output for a few days before attending a urology clinic.

Your appointment at the flow clinic will probably last two to three hours, and you will be told to drink plenty of fluid before you arrive at the hospital so that your bladder is full. On arrival, you will be asked to provide a sample of urine to be checked for infection. There are several diagnostic tests which can be done to determine the cause of your problem and you may have some or all of them. If you are likely to need an operation, you may also have a chest X-ray to assess your general fitness for surgery.

Urine flow test

You will be asked to drink more water and, when your bladder is full again, to pass urine into a special funnel-shaped container with a meter attached. The meter measures the volume of urine you pass and its rate of flow, and records the measurements on a chart. A low flow rate may indicate obstruction of the bladder or urethra, and a low volume that urine is being retained in the bladder. This test may be repeated once or twice when you have drunk more water.

Ultrasound test

You may be given an ultrasound scan after each passage of urine. Ultrasound (also called ultrasonography) involves passing high-frequency sound waves through the body wall. When the sound waves encounter a solid object, they are reflected back like an echo and can be processed by a computer to build up an image which is displayed on a screen. A small scanning device will be passed over your lower abdomen and any enlargement or abnormality of the prostate, or any residual urine left in the bladder, will be apparent. The procedure is completely painless. If there is no ultrasound machine at your urology clinic, you may be given an appointment for a scan to be done in an X-ray department at a later date.

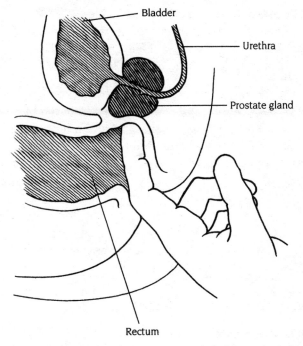

Bladder

Urethra

Prostate gland

Rectum

Rectal examination. The doctor inserts a gloved finger into the rectum to feel the prostate gland.

Rectal examination

As the prostate gland is close to the rectum, it can be felt during a manual rectal examination, done before or after the flow tests. A doctor will insert a gloved finger into your rectum and should be able to feel whether your prostate is hard, enlarged or nodular. A large, smooth prostate indicates a benign condition, whereas a harder, nodular one may be a sign of prostate cancer. This is not a very sensitive test and whatever its outcome you will require further evaluation.

Blood tests

A sample of your blood may be taken so that the levels of two substances can be measured and possibly also to assess your kidney function.

Prostate specific antigen (PSA) is a protein produced by the normal prostate. Although it is always present in the blood, its level increases with increasing age, size of the prostate and in prostatitis. A significantly raised level of PSA may indicate the presence of prostate cancer. However, the measurement has to be viewed in the context of other symptoms and signs, and further tests will always be done to clarify the findings.

The level of another blood component, prostatic acid phosphatase (PAP), sometimes increases when prostate cancer develops, although its measurement is now considered to be of limited use as a diagnostic tool.

Intravenous urogram/pyelogram

Urograms (also known as pyelograms) provide an outline of the entire urinary tract and are sometimes done to examine the kidneys if there is blood in the urine. If you have a urogram, it will be done in the X-ray department and will take about an hour to complete.

A simple X-ray will be taken before a contrast agent is injected into a vein in your arm. After an hour or so, the contrast agent (which is like a dye) will start to be excreted by your kidneys and will pass through the ureters and bladder, at which time a further series of X-rays will be taken. Apart from showing the size and shape of the kidneys, the X-rays will also highlight any defects in the urinary system, such as the presence of stones or tumours, and may show up any abnormalities in the bladder and, occasionally, in the prostate.

FURTHER TESTS

If there is any doubt about the cause of your prostate problems after your visit to the flow clinic, or if cancer is suspected, you may be asked to return for further tests.

Transrectal ultrasound scanning (TRUS)

This procedure involves the insertion of an ultrasound probe into the rectum to take pictures of the prostate, which lies along the front rectal wall. You will probably be asked to lie on your

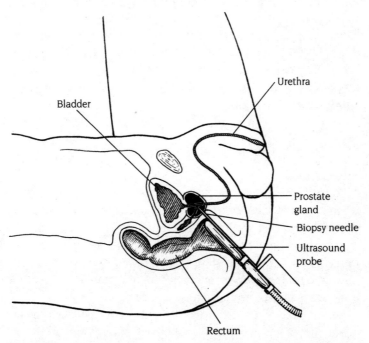

An ultrasound probe. The probe is inserted through the rectum and guides the biopsy needle to the correct position for a sample of tissue to be taken from the prostate gland.

left side with your knees drawn up against your chest as the ultrasound probe is inserted. The probe is lubricated with a jelly and covered with a condom to keep it clean, and will be moved up and down within the rectum to produce two-dimensional pictures of your prostate, bladder and surrounding areas.

The scan takes about 10 to 15 minutes, and is usually done in an investigation room in the out-patients' department or day theatre area.

Prostate biopsy

A biopsy is often performed at the same time as a transrectal ultrasound scan to obtain tissue from the prostate to make a diagnosis or to detect or exclude prostate cancer.

The biopsy needle is usually inserted into the rectum and through the front part of the rectal wall into the prostate gland. The least uncomfortable, and most accurate, way of doing this biopsy is to pass the needle down a special channel alongside the ultrasound probe.

You will be given an antibiotic injection (and possibly antibiotic tablets to take for a few days afterwards). Despite these precautions, it is still possible for infection to develop after a prostate biopsy.

Four to six samples of tissue are usually taken at one time when cancer is suspected. The biopsy specimens will be sent to the pathology laboratory for examination. It may take several working days before the results are available. If the biopsy confirms the presence of prostate cancer, further tests such as computerised tomography, magnetic resonance imaging and isotope bone scans may be arranged for you (see below).

Because the biopsy involves cutting the tissue of the prostate gland, there may be blood in your bowel motions and urine for a day or so afterwards. As 40 per cent of the content of semen comes from the prostate, your semen may also contain blood, which may persist for several weeks.

Chest X-ray

If prostate cancer is suspected, a chest X-ray may be taken to determine whether it has spread to the lungs, although this is not a common site for metastases.

Isotope bone scan

A bone scan may be done to detect any secondary tumours in your skeleton. A small dose of a radioactive isotope will be injected into a vein in your arm and you will be able to leave the out-patients' department for two to three hours while it is taken up by the bones. (The amount of radioactivity involved is no more than that of a conventional kidney X-ray.)

When you return, you will be asked to lie on a table while a special scanning camera is passed over your body. Although the isotope is taken up by normal bone, more is absorbed by areas of cancer, which will show up as patches on the scan. The whole of your skeleton will be scanned, with particular attention being paid to your spine, pelvis and ribs. The procedure takes 30 to 45 minutes.

Computerised tomography (CT)

Computerised tomography is another way of producing a picture of the prostate and surrounding structures. It is done to look for regional spread of prostate cancer to the lymph nodes. You may be given an injection of a contrast agent as well as some to drink. You will then be asked to lie on a table which passes through a large hoop-shaped scanner while X-rays are taken which are interpreted by a computer.

Magnetic resonance imaging (MRI)

Like computerised tomography, magnetic resonance imaging is another form of body scan done to detect spread of cancer to the regional lymph nodes. However, it does not involve the use of X-rays and the scanner in this case is a large, high-powered magnet. Following the injection of a contrast medium, you will be asked to lie on a table which will pass through a tunnel containing the magnet. Again, a picture of the prostate gland and nearby structures is produced by a computer.

Some people are unable to tolerate the whole scan because the tunnel makes them claustrophobic. As the procedure involves the use of a magnet, you must not take anything metal into the scanning tunnel.

Staging of prostate cancer   Staging of a cancer allows an assessment to be made of how far it has spread, if at all. The stage at which it is first detected will determine what treatment is most likely to be effective. Localised cancer which has not spread beyond the prostate gland can sometimes be cured by major surgery. Surgery is not appropriate for local spread outside the capsule or for regional spread to the pelvic lymph nodes, and treatment with radiotherapy may be recommended in these cases. Although advanced cancer with metastases at distant sites around the body cannot be cured, treatment is available in the form of hormone therapy.

Staging will involve some of the tests described above:

* digital rectal examination to feel the prostate gland,
* transrectal ultrasound,
* measurement of the level of prostate specific antigen in the blood which will indicate broadly whether the cancer is localised or has spread to distant parts of the body,
* magnetic resonance imaging,
* computerised tomography,
* isotope bone scanning to look for spread to the bones.

DISCUSSIONS AND DECISIONS

Whether or not you are seen by a urologist during your visit to the clinic, you are likely to have an appointment with one at some time to discuss the results of your tests and the possible courses of action.

Depending on your test results and on various other factors, the urologist will advise you of the best treatment for your prostate problem. Do ask any questions, and bear in mind that the final decision to have a particular treatment is yours. You may want to ask for time to discuss things with your partner or other family members. You may not take in all you are told by the doctor at this time but the hospital may have a clinical nurse specialist or nurse practitioner who can talk to you and your partner to explain your diagnosis and any proposed treatment in more detail. Even if there is no nurse specialist at the clinic, there should be a nurse available with particular experience and knowledge of urology who can explain things to you. So do ask if you would like to talk to someone and if you need explanations of anything you have not understood.

There are possible side-effects related to prostate surgery, and these should be explained clearly to you before you make the decision to go ahead with treatment.

CHAPTER 3

Treatment options

The choice of treatment depends on various factors, including the cause of your prostate problem, the degree of severity of any symptoms, your age and state of general health. This chapter briefly describes the different types of treatment available for benign and malignant prostate conditions. Details of the surgical procedures are given in Chapter 6, and of non-surgical treatments for prostate cancer in Chapters 9 and 10. The treatment of prostatitis, which is invariably with drugs, has already been discussed on page 7.

BENIGN PROSTATIC HYPERPLASIA

There are various treatment options to relieve the symptoms of benign prostate enlargement. In some cases the situation can be monitored and further action need only be considered if the symptoms worsen and become troublesome.

Watchful waiting

When an enlarged prostate causes mild to moderate urinary symptoms, or if symptoms are severe but surgery is contraindicated, for example because of poor general health, watchful waiting may be appropriate. Treatment for benign prostatic enlargement is aimed at relieving symptoms and there is no evidence that it is needed to prevent further problems in later life. The majority of men with mild to moderate symptoms will experience no worsening of their condition, and sometimes symptoms improve spontaneously in time. Therefore watchful waiting is a safe and reasonable option in these cases.

You may be seen regularly by your family doctor or urologist, possibly every six months, so that your condition can be monitored, or you may be told to contact your doctor if your symptoms worsen.

Drug treatment

Moderate symptoms of benign prostatic enlargement which are not severe enough to warrant surgery can sometimes be relieved by drugs.

There are two main groups of drugs appropriate in cases of obstruction. First are the *alpha blockers* (for example indoramin and alfuzosin) which block the alpha nerve receptors in the prostate and often improve symptoms considerably. They sometimes induce side-effects of a dry mouth and light-headedness. The second group comprises the 5 *alpha-reductase inhibitors* (for example finasteride) which can make the prostate shrink by up to 30 per cent by interfering with the action of the hormones which make it grow. It may be about six months before you experience any real benefit from these drugs, and they are not generally as effective as the alpha blockers. They can also affect the ability to obtain an erection and cannot be tolerated by some men.

For irritative symptoms due to bladder instability, such as frequency or urgency, *anticholinergic* drugs (for example oxybutynin) may be effective. However, irritative symptoms secondary to obstruction caused by prostate enlargement can be made worse by anticholinergics and can occasionally lead to urinary retention.

Stents

A stent is a small, coiled or spiral device, usually made of steel or titanium, which can be inserted to lie in the urethra at the point where it is surrounded by the prostate. It keeps the lobes of the prostate apart, relieving any obstruction and allowing normal micturition. The stent is inserted under local or general anaesthetic using an instrument called a **cystoscope**. A cystoscope comprises a telescope and an attachment for a light source; other surgical instruments can be inserted through its core.

Stents can move out of position and give rise to stones. They are less effective than surgery and are only really an option for older men whose general health is poor and for whom an operation would be inadvisable.

Surgery

If you have troublesome symptoms, or even if you have mild symptoms but tests show that you have an enlarged prostate which may cause urine retention and eventually affect the function of your kidneys, you may be advised to have an operation called a **prostatectomy**. There are various types of prostatectomy, but all involve the removal of some or all of the prostate tissue. Studies in different countries indicate that there is a 10 to 20 per cent chance of a 50-year-old man requiring a prostatectomy during his lifetime.

In most cases, a prostatectomy reduces symptoms, although it is not always successful and can occasionally cause side-effects. The surgeon should discuss the possible side-effects with you and you should consider them carefully before you opt for surgical treatment. The most common post-operative complications are discussed in Chapter 8.

Transurethral resection of the prostate (TURP)
The vast majority of prostatectomies are done through the urethra using a general or spinal anaesthetic (see Chapter 5). Prostate tissue is removed using an instrument called a **resec-**

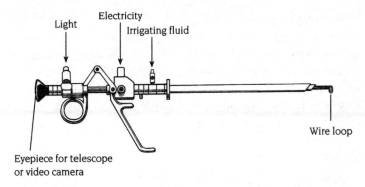

A resectoscope.

toscope through which an electric current is passed to produce heat in a wire loop at its tip. The loop is used to chip away the prostate tissue obstructing the urethra. The pieces of prostate tissue fall back into the bladder and are washed out through the penis and sent to the laboratory to be examined under a microscope for any signs of cancer.

The operation takes about 45 minutes or less and, as it does not involve any cutting of the wall of the abdomen (and therefore no wounds or scar), recovery is relatively rapid, although the cut surfaces of the prostate will need time to heal.

Open prostatectomy

An open prostatectomy may be done on an extremely large prostate or when there is an associated problem such as a large bladder stone which needs to be removed at the same time. A spinal or general anaesthetic is used (or very occasionally an epidural) and the operation is performed through an incision made in the abdominal wall. Once the prostate gland has been removed, the incision is closed with stitches. The recovery period is longer than that following a transurethral resection as the abdominal wound and bladder have to heal.

Bladder neck incision

A bladder neck incision may be done to improve the flow of urine. A cut may be made in the neck of the bladder, leaving the prostate intact, or along the whole length of the prostate itself, an operation sometimes known as a **prostatotomy**. A bladder neck incision can relieve the symptoms caused by a smaller prostate, for which it is as effective as a transurethral resection (see above).

Laser and microwave treatments

These new techniques are basically designed to heat, and thereby shrink, the prostate. They are sometimes used as alternatives to transurethral resection to treat benign prostate conditions (not cancer) and to relieve symptoms of bladder outflow obstruction. However, they are not widely available at the present time, although clinical trials (see p.31) are currently underway in many areas to assess their efficacy.

Microwave treatment

Microwave treatment involves the use of microwave radiation to heat selected areas of prostate tissue to a temperature at which the cells die and the tissue is destroyed. The microwaves can be delivered via a catheter inserted through the urethra and into the prostate gland, or through the rectal wall via a probe inserted into the rectum. Local anaesthetic is sometimes used, although the procedure may be done without anaesthesia. The treatment may need to be repeated.

Although microwave treatment is quite effective in relieving symptoms, its long-term efficacy has not yet been established. Like laser treatment, it does not cause any bleeding or any of the other possible side-effects of surgery.

Laser treatment

Lasers are a form of energy which can be used to shrink the

prostate gland. The energy is delivered via a cystoscope (see p.28) inserted through the penis and into the prostate. The procedure normally requires the use of a general or spinal anaesthetic, although local anaesthesia is occasionally used. This type of treatment is currently under evaluation.

Clinical trials   To be able to improve the treatment given to men with prostate disease, new therapies need to be tested, and currently used drugs and treatment regimes need to be tried in different ways. Therefore men are sometimes asked to take part in clinical trials to compare a new treatment with an existing one.

If your doctor is involved in a trial of this sort, you may be asked if you would be willing to take part. The details of the trial will be explained to you, and you should make sure you fully understand what is entailed before you make a decision. You are under no obligation to agree to be involved and if you refuse, the quality of the treatment you receive will not be affected in any way.

PROSTATE CANCER

The treatment for prostate cancer will depend to a large extent on its stage (see p.24) and on whether it has already spread by the time it is first detected.

Watchful waiting

For a small, slow-growing prostate cancer in an older man or in a younger man who has mild or no symptoms, watchful waiting may be the treatment of choice. The cancer will be monitored at regular check-ups so that any signs of change can be detected. If you experience any deterioration in your condition between check-ups, you should let your doctor know immediately rather than waiting for your next appointment.

Surgery

Radical prostatectomy

A small cancer in the early stages of development which is confined to the prostate may be treated by the removal of the entire prostate gland, its capsule and the seminal vesicles. The operation is performed through a long, vertical incision in the abdominal wall. It is major surgery which is most suitable for the treatment of younger, fitter men and there is currently debate as to whether its use is ever justified in older men.

Orchidectomy

Very occasionally, the testes are surgically removed to reduce the body's production of the male hormone testosterone on which prostate cancer depends. Therefore, although it is a surgical procedure, orchidectomy is strictly speaking a form of hormone therapy. It may control a prostate cancer at an advanced stage, although it cannot cure it.

Pelvic node dissection

Also called **lymphadenectomy**, this procedure is sometimes done at the same time as prostate surgery. The lymph nodes in the pelvis are removed so that they can be examined for signs of regional spread of the cancer. If metastases are discovered in the lymph nodes, the surgeon will not proceed to radical surgery as an operation cannot effect a cure once spread has occurred. In some hospitals, the lymph nodes are removed laparoscopically (by 'keyhole surgery') several weeks before radical surgery is scheduled so that they can be examined histologically and a decision made as to whether or not to proceed.

There is no evidence to suggest that pelvic node dissection is itself therapeutic, but it is sometimes a useful tool in staging a prostate cancer before deciding on the most suitable treatment.

Radiotherapy

Instead of radical surgery, radiotherapy is sometimes the primary treatment for younger men with localised prostate cancer or in the very early stages of local spread. It can also help relieve pain due to secondary tumours in the bones, in which case it may be given at the same time as hormone therapy or if pain recurs after hormone therapy has stopped (see p.87). Occasionally, treatment has to be repeated.

Details of radiotherapy are given in Chapter 9.

Hormone therapy

There are various hormonal treatments for advanced prostate cancer. They all work by taking away the male hormone drive to the cancer cells, thereby reducing the growth of the tumour, sometimes for many years. Apart from the surgical removal of the testes (see p.32), hormone therapy includes the use of various drugs which mimic the effects of certain of the body's own hormones. It is often used as a long-term treatment.

Hormone therapy is described in more detail in Chapter 10.

Chemotherapy

Drugs are sometimes used to treat cancers which have spread to other parts of the body. However, this type of therapy is rarely used in the treatment of prostate cancer, particularly in Britain, as it tends not to be very effective.

CHAPTER 4

Going in to hospital for an operation

This chapter explains what is likely to happen if you are admitted to a National Health Service (NHS) hospital in the UK, but the procedures are broadly the same for private care too (see Chapter 11).

You should receive a letter from the hospital telling you the date of your operation and any other details you need to know, and possibly also a leaflet explaining the admission procedures and what to take in with you. If you have been put on a shortlist and an operating slot becomes available unexpectedly, you may be telephoned and asked to come in at short notice, possibly within a day or two.

A few days before you are admitted to hospital for surgery, you may be asked to attend a **pre-admission clerking clinic**. During this clinic, a doctor will explain your operation and answer any questions you may have. Any necessary pre-operative tests may also be done so that the results are available by the time you enter hospital for your operation. You may also be asked to sign a consent form at this time (see p.44).

The time of your admission depends on the normal practice at your particular hospital. If you have already had a pre-clerking appointment, you may be able to enter hospital on the day of your operation. Otherwise you will be admitted the day before so that the tests can be done and the results received.

You will probably be in hospital for two to three days following a transurethral resection, and for five to seven days following an open or radical prostatectomy. Day-case surgery is not appropriate for any type of prostate operation, although it is occasionally possible to leave hospital the day after a bladder neck incision.

WHAT TO TAKE IN TO HOSPITAL

1 *Nightclothes*. You will be given a hospital gown to wear during your operation but should take your own nightclothes to put on when you are back on the ward. You will also need slippers and a dressing gown.

2 *Towel and washing things*.

3 *Money*. A *small* amount of money may be useful for newspapers and the telephone. Large sums of money and wallets should not be taken into hospital as these may have to be kept in an unlocked cabinet by your bed. If you have to take any valuables or large sums of money with you, they should be given to the ward sister for safe keeping when you are admitted. You will be given a receipt listing each item and should keep this safe so that you can collect your possessions when you are discharged. However, hospital authorities strongly discourage people from bringing anything of great value with them unless absolutely necessary. It is better to make arrangements for any valuables you do not wish to leave at home to be looked after by a relative or friend while you are in hospital.

4 *Books, magazines, puzzles etc*. There will inevitably be periods of waiting between visits from medical staff before your operation, and you may want something to occupy you during this time as well as post-operatively.

5 *Drugs you are already taking*. Once your admission has been arranged, your family doctor will have been asked to fill in a form stating all the drugs you are taking and their doses. You may be asked to take your drugs with you when you are

admitted to hospital so that their dosages can be checked and so that you can continue to be given any which are necessary. All your drugs will be kept for you during your stay as you must only take those which are given to you by medical staff. They should, however, be returned to you before you leave.

6   *Admission letter*. You should take with you the admission letter sent to you from the hospital.

Wedding rings   Wedding rings, or any other rings which are very precious to you or which cannot be removed, will be covered with adhesive tape before your operation. This is to prevent the metal causing burns during the process of **electrocautery** which is used to control bleeding during surgery. In electrocautery an electric current heats the tip of an instrument which is used to shrivel and seal the little blood vessels and stop them bleeding.

HOSPITAL STAFF

The ward of a hospital is a busy place and can seem rather confusing and frightening. It may help to have an idea of the different medical staff you are likely to meet, and the jobs they do.

Nurses

The uniforms worn to distinguish nurses of different ranks will vary from hospital to hospital, but all nurses wear badges which state clearly their name and sometimes their grade. There are, of course, both male and female nurses, although women are still in the majority. The nursing grades are as follows.

1   The most senior nurse on the ward is the *ward sister* or *ward manager*. Each ward will have one ward sister who will be very

experienced and able to answer any questions you may have. The ward sister has 24-hour a day responsibility for all the staff and patients on at least one ward, for the day-to-day running of the ward, standards of care etc., and is ultimately responsible for the ward even when not on duty. She will be a registered nurse (RN) or a registered general nurse (RGN), who has usually been qualified for at least five years. Ward sisters may wear a uniform of a single colour, often dark blue.

The male equivalent of the ward sister is a *charge nurse*, whose rank will be clearly displayed on his name badge. Charge nurses wear a white tunic.

2   When the ward sister is not on duty, there may be a *senior staff nurse* or a *team leader* of another grade in charge. The senior staff nurse is deputy to, and works closely with, the ward sister. Like the ward sister, this nurse will be very experienced.

3   Each ward may have several *staff nurses* – registered or registered general nurses who have completed their nursing training. They may be newly qualified or may have several years' experience, and will take charge of the ward when both the ward sister and senior staff nurse are unavailable. There are different grades of staff nurse, distinguished by different coloured belts, epaulettes, uniforms or, more rarely nowadays, hats.

The more junior staff nurses are very often in their first or second post since qualifying. They are less involved in ward management, and are therefore able to work closely with the patients.

4   *Enrolled nurses* have undergone two years of training. They are gradually being replaced and can now undergo a training programme to become staff nurses with the qualification RGN. However, there are still many enrolled nurses working on hospital wards who are very experienced and sometimes team leaders (see above).

5   As student nurses now spend more time in college and less on the wards of hospitals, *health care assistants* (HCAs) are being brought in to take their place. These are unqualified nurses who have undergone six months' training on day release while working on a ward and who have then been assessed for a National Vocational Qualification (NVQ) by senior nurses. Health care assistants are able to carry out all basic nursing duties except for the dispensing of drugs. They are supervised at all times by a qualified nurse.

6   The ward may also have several *nursing auxiliaries* who are present to deal with any non-medical jobs and to help with the basic care of patients such as making beds, serving tea, and putting away linen etc. Although nursing auxiliaries are not trained nurses, some are very experienced and have acquired greater responsibility.

7   Student nurses – *diploma nursing students* or *Project* 2000 *students* – are unpaid and allocated to the wards at various stages during their college-based training. They are mainly involved in observing and carrying out limited clinical tasks. In their last term before they qualify, they will be rostered on to nursing shifts and be part of a ward team.

Doctors

Each consultant surgeon in a hospital may head a team of doctors of different ranks, sometimes known as a 'firm'. You may meet some or all of them. These doctors can, of course, be men or women.

1   The *consultant surgeon* holds the ultimate responsibility for all the patients on the operating list, and for the work of all the staff in the 'firm'. Consultants have at least 10 to 15 years' experience as surgeons.

Unless you are being treated privately, you may not actually see the consultant who is responsible for your care, but should be visited on the ward before your operation by whichever surgeon is to perform it.

2   The *senior registrar* is a very experienced surgeon who has completed several years of training and will soon be appointed to a consultant post. However, this grade of surgeon is soon to be changed.

3   Your operation may be performed by a *registrar* rather than by a consultant surgeon or senior registrar. Registrars have trained as surgeons for at least two or three years and are able to carry out some surgery alone, assisting the consultant, or being assisted by the consultant, on more difficult operations.

4   Some hospitals employ *clinical assistants* as surgeons. These are often very experienced surgeons who, for personal or family reasons, are not able to work full time.

5   You may be examined before your operation by a *senior house officer* (SHO) or by a house surgeon (see below). Senior house officers have been qualified doctors for between one and five years, and are gaining further experience in hospital before becoming surgeons or specialising in another branch of medicine.

6   A *house surgeon* (or *house officer*) is likely to be directly concerned with your care both before and after your operation, taking notes of your medical history and arranging for any necessary pre-operative investigations to be done, such as a blood count, chest X-ray or electrocardiogram. House officers are qualified doctors who have completed at least five years of undergraduate training and are working for a further year in hospital before becoming fully registered. Although house officers do not perform surgery on their own, they may assist the surgeon in the operating theatre.

Anaesthetists are doctors who have been trained in the administration of drugs which cause loss of sensation or consciousness, or both (anaesthetics) and those which block feelings of pain (analgesics). An anaesthetist may visit you before your operation to discuss any relevant details, such as any anaesthetics you have had in the past and any drugs you may be taking (see Chapter 5), and will be present throughout your operation.

Medical social workers

If any problems arise at home during your stay in hospital, or if you are concerned about being able to manage on your own once you return home, you can ask to talk to a medical social worker. Medical social workers work in close partnership with other medical staff in the hospital and will be able to give you advice and practical support. If necessary, you may be kept in hospital a little longer until nursing staff are happy that you will be able to manage or that arrangements have been made to help you once you are at home. 'Meals on wheels' or a home help should be available for anyone who needs them.

BEFORE THE OPERATION

The following gives a general idea of what is likely to happen once you are admitted to the ward, although procedures do vary a little from hospital to hospital.

Admission to the ward

When you arrive at the hospital, you should report to the main reception desk with your admission letter. The staff there will check your details and tell you which ward to go to. Once on the ward, the ward clerk or a nurse will deal with the clerical side of your admission, filling in the necessary forms with you. You will then be shown to your bed and told of any ward details such as meal times, where to find the toilets, day room etc.

In Britain, the Government's Patients' Charter introduced the 'Named Nurse Initiative'. Each patient in an NHS hospital is allocated a **named nurse** who is responsible for planning that patient's nursing care throughout their stay. The ward sister will, of course, still be informed of all aspects of your care, and will be able to discuss it with you or your relatives.

Your named nurse will admit you to the ward, look after you during your stay, and co-ordinate your discharge when the time comes. Other nurses will be allocated from the team for other working shifts. The idea is for people to be identified as individuals who are known to at least one nurse on each shift and who are involved in their own care. To this end, you may be asked to help your nurse draw up a care plan when you are admitted to the ward. You should tell the nurse of any ailments, preferences or dislikes you have, for example if you prefer to sleep with several pillows or if there are certain foods you do not want.

Your nurse's name may be displayed above your bed or on your bedside locker so that your relatives and other nursing and medical staff know who to talk to about your care. Your care plan may be kept at the bottom of your bed, but wherever it is, it is available for you to read. Nursing staff may tick off a checklist as they carry out the various procedures and will update the care plan with you as the need arises.

The nurse will measure your blood pressure, temperature and pulse. A sample of your urine may be taken for analysis and you may be weighed as the anaesthetist may need to know your weight in order to be able to calculate the dose of anaesthetic you require.

When your discharge is planned the nursing staff will need to be sure that someone will be able to collect you and take you home when the time comes. If this is not possible, hospital transport may be arranged for you.

Do tell a nurse if you have any problems or if you are anxious about *any* aspect of your hospital stay.

Anti-embolism stockings

Once you are settled on the ward, a nurse may measure your legs for anti-embolism stockings (often called TEDS –**t**hrombo-**e**mbolic **d**eterrent **s**tockings) to wear during your operation and until you are mobile afterwards. These stockings are used routinely in some hospitals, and are almost always worn by anyone having a radical prostatectomy for which the period of post-operative immobility may be slightly longer than for other types of prostate surgery. Although they may feel uncomfortable, particularly when the weather is hot, there is no doubt as to their value.

Normally, the activity of the muscles in the legs helps to keep the blood moving through them. During long periods of bed rest or anaesthesia, these muscles are inactive and the circulation of blood in the legs slows down. A blood clot (**thrombus**) is thus more likely to form which can block the passage of blood through the vein, causing **thrombosis**. If a piece of this clot breaks off, it forms an **embolus** which, if it travels through the circulation and lodges in a vital organ such as the lung, can cause **pulmonary embolism**, with serious consequences. Anti-embolism stockings help prevent blood clots forming in the deep veins of the legs by improving the venous return to the heart.

A nurse will measure your calf and thigh and the length of your leg, and will give you a pair of stockings of the correct size. If you have a history of varicose veins or thrombosis which increases your risk of developing a blood clot, you will probably have to wear the stockings throughout your hospital stay.

Otherwise you may not need to put them on until you are preparing to go to the operating theatre and will be able to remove them once you are up and about again after your operation.

Heparin injections

If you are having a radical prostatectomy, have a history of thrombosis, or are otherwise at high risk of developing blood clots, you will be given low-dose heparin injections during your stay in hospital. Heparin is an anticoagulant which occurs naturally in the body, thinning the blood and preventing it from clotting. The use of low-dose heparin may also be advised for men having a transurethral resection of the prostate.

Visit by a doctor

As has already been mentioned, a house surgeon or senior house officer will visit you on the ward before your operation to take details of your medical history – including any allergies you may have and any drugs you are taking – and to examine you. Your family doctor may have already filled in a form giving the names and dosages of any drugs you have been prescribed, and you should have been told what to do about these. Do not forget to tell the hospital doctor of any other drugs you have been taking which your family doctor may not be aware of, such as vitamin supplements, cough medicines, aspirins etc., which are available from a pharmacy without the need for prescription.

A medical examination will be carried out to identify any illness or infection you may have which could complicate the use of a general anaesthetic. If you are over 50 years of age or a heavy smoker, you will probably have a chest X-ray and an electrocardiogram so that any potential anaesthetic complications due to breathing or heart problems can be picked up.

The surgeon who is to perform your operation may also visit you on the ward to check that all is well.

Consent forms

Either at a pre-operative clinic visit or before you sign the consent form, you will be told about the possible risks associated with prostate operations, such as urinary incontinence and impotence (see p.78). By signing the consent form you are declaring that your operation has been explained to you and that you understand what it entails and have agreed to it taking place. You are also giving your permission for the doctors to take whatever action they feel to be appropriate should some emergency occur during surgery, and for any necessary anaesthetic to be given to you. Do read this form carefully, and ask the doctor to explain anything you do not understand.

Visit by the anaesthetist

The anaesthetist will probably come to see you to discuss anything that may be relevant to the choice of anaesthetic given to you.

Anaesthetics have improved considerably during the last few years, and a 'pre-med.' is now not always given routinely. If you or your anaesthetist feel that you are very anxious and need something to relax you, you may be given some form of pre-med. two or three hours before the operation to sedate you. If you enter hospital the day before your operation and think that you will be too anxious to sleep that night, you can ask the house surgeon or senior house officer for something to help you.

False teeth

You should tell the anaesthetist if you have any false teeth or dental bridges as these will have to be removed before you go into the operating theatre. A broken or loose tooth can be inhaled into the lungs during surgery. You should also point out any teeth which are crowned. At some hospitals you will be able to wear your false teeth until you reach the operating theatre rather than having to take them out on the ward.

'Nil by mouth'

This is a term which means that neither food nor drink must be swallowed. In order to prevent vomiting and the risk of choking on your vomit while you are anaesthetised, you will be told not to eat or drink anything for four to six hours before an operation done using a general anaesthetic, although you will be able to have a few sips of water with any tablets you need to take. If you are admitted the night before surgery, you will be able to have supper on the ward. If you enter hospital in the morning and your operation is to be that afternoon, you should not eat or drink for about six hours beforehand. However, some anaesthetists now allow their patients to drink clear fluids up to three hours pre-operatively.

Shaving

Just before an open or radical prostatectomy your lower abdomen, groin and scrotum will have to be shaved. This is done to reduce the risk of infection and to give the surgeon a clear view of the area to be operated on. It also makes the changing or removal of the adhesive wound covering less painful.

You may be given a disposable razor or possibly clippers to shave yourself, or it may be done by a nurse. If you are anxious about doing it yourself, or have arthritis in your hands or some other condition which would make shaving difficult, do ask a nurse to do it for you.

Smoking

If you are a heavy smoker and have not been able to cut down or stop altogether, you will be advised not to smoke in the hours before your operation. It is, of course, much better to stop smoking some months before surgery. The carbon monoxide contained in cigarette smoke poisons the blood by replacing some of the oxygen which is carried in it and which is vital to processes such as wound healing.

Obesity

Obesity adds to the risk of general anaesthesia, and for this reason people who are very overweight should try to lose weight before entering hospital. Some surgeons are reluctant to carry out non-emergency operations on heavy smokers or obese patients as they consider the risks to be too great. However, starting a long, strict diet before your operation may also be inadvisable. The consultant will have assessed your weight during your out-patients appointment, and will probably have given you some guidance at that time.

Waiting

It may seem that you have been admitted to hospital unnecessarily early, and you may find you have to wait on the ward with little to do. Apart from having to be seen by all the medical staff mentioned above, who are responsible for many other patients as well, time will also have been allowed for the assessment of any medical problems you may have, and for the results of blood tests etc. to be received.

Sometimes surgery has to be cancelled at the last moment if an emergency has arisen and an earlier operation has taken longer than expected. Although this would be distressing, it would only occur if an operation taking place before your own had met with complications. If so, you will probably be sent home and called again at the earliest opportunity. Do try not to get upset. Other operations taking place on the same day may be more urgent than yours and cannot be postponed. Under the terms of the Patients' Charter, a cancelled operation must be done within one month.

As surgery taking place before yours may take longer than expected, you will probably be given only an approximate time for your operation, being told if it is scheduled for the morning or afternoon.

Leaving the ward for your operation

Before being taken from the ward to the anaesthetic room or operating theatre, you will be given a hospital operating gown to wear, and a plastic-covered bracelet bearing your name and an identifying hospital number will be attached to one or both of your wrists. You will then leave the ward on a hospital trolley.

The anaesthetic room

In the anaesthetic room, a small tube called a **cannula** will be inserted into a vein in the back of your hand. The cannula will be kept in place throughout the operation and provides a channel for the administration of drugs. The anaesthetic will probably be administered in the anaesthetic room, although it may be given in the operating theatre itself.

Once the anaesthetic has taken effect, which will happen within seconds, you are ready for your operation.

CHAPTER 5

Anaesthesia for surgery

The anaesthetic chosen for you will depend largely on the type of operation you are having and on the normal practice of your anaesthetist. It may be possible for your own preferences to be taken into account, if you have any, so do discuss them with the anaesthetist during the ward visit.

LOCAL ANAESTHESIA

Occasionally, a local anaesthetic is used for transurethral resection of the prostate. The anaesthetic is injected either through a cystoscope into the prostate itself or around the prostate to block the nerves. You will probably also be given a sedative to put you to sleep. This type of anaesthesia is not commonly used in Britain, although it is current practice in some other countries.

SPINAL ANAESTHESIA

A spinal anaesthetic is a type of regional anaesthetic which is injected between the vertebrae of the spine into the space around the nerves in the back. It causes numbness below the waist which lasts for three to five hours, thus giving effective pain relief for a period after the operation is over.

You may also be given a sedative to make you drowsy. Once the anaesthetic has been injected into your back, it will take effect after five to ten minutes, causing your legs and lower body to become numb and heavy.

Epidural anaesthesia

Epidural anaesthetics are similar to spinal anaesthetics and are occasionally used for some types of prostate surgery, usually radical prostatectomies. A tube is inserted into the back, close to the nerves leaving the spine, through which pain-killing drugs are injected at a slow, constant rate. Epidurals provide excellent pain relief and are sometimes left in place for several days after an operation.

GENERAL ANAESTHESIA

General anaesthesia can be used for all types of prostate operations. A general anaesthetic will put you to sleep so that you have no feeling in any part of your body. It may be an **intravenous anaesthetic**, injected into a vein in your hand or arm through a plastic tube, or an **inhalational anaesthetic** in the form of a gas which you breathe in. In fact, both types are normally used, although you will probably only be aware of the injection which sends you off to sleep.

If you are having a general anaesthetic, you may be visited by an anaesthetist on the ward before your operation (see p.44). The main reason for this visit is to decide what type of anaesthesia would be safest for you. It also gives you the opportunity to discuss any problems or worries you may have. The anaesthetist will ask you several questions about any anaesthetics you have had before, any drugs you are taking, and about your general health. It is important that you answer these questions as fully as possible. You should also mention to the anaesthetist if you have any false or crowned teeth (see p.44).

If you have had problems in the past such as an allergy to a particular anaesthetic, it will be helpful if you know the name of the drug concerned or the hospital where the operation was carried out. The appropriate records can then be checked to make sure another type of anaesthetic is used. You should also tell the anaesthetist if you know of any other member of your family who has reacted against a particular drug, as you may have the same problem.

Risks of general anaesthesia

People with certain medical conditions, such as serious heart or lung disease, may not be given general anaesthetics as they are potentially at greater risk.

Some people are afraid of being put to sleep by a general anaesthetic, but the risk is small (see p.79). If you are worried about it, do discuss it with the anaesthetist.

Other medication

The anaesthetist will explain about other tablets and drugs which may be required before your operation. You may be given the option of having pre-medication (a 'pre-med.'), usually in the form of tablets given one to two hours before surgery. If you are anxious about your operation, you may wish to ask for a 'pre-med.' if their use is not routine in your hospital.

If there is a reason for you to have antibiotics or blood thinning drugs, this will also be explained to you by the anaesthetist. You may be given any drugs which you normally take, such as diuretics ('water tablets') or drugs to reduce high blood pressure.

Before your operation

You will probably be told not to have anything to eat or drink for about six hours before the operation ('nil by mouth'). The reason for this is that any food or drink left in your stomach could cause you to be sick while you are under the influence of the anaesthetic. However, this practice is gradually changing, and in many cases it is possible to take clear fluids up to four or even two hours before surgery.

If you are having a 'pre-med.', it will be given to you on the ward, and you will soon begin to feel sleepy. There is no need to be alarmed: the 'pre-med.' is not an anaesthetic itself, it is only to relax you so that you are not anxious before the operation.

When the time comes to take you to the operating theatre, you will be asked several questions to confirm your identity and to make sure that you are ready for surgery. These questions may be repeated several times by different people: many people have many types of operations each day in a hospital and checks are essential to make sure no mistakes are made.

When you are taken from the ward, you may go first to the anaesthetic room or straight to the operating theatre to be given your anaesthetic. The anaesthetist, or an assistant, will fit some monitoring devices to watch over you while you are asleep. These may include a little probe which goes on your finger to measure the amount of oxygen in your blood, an electrocardiogram (ECG) to observe your heart beat, and a cuff around your arm to measure your blood pressure. A cannula will be put into a vein in the back of your hand or arm, and the anaesthetic drugs will be introduced into your body through it. Once the anaesthetist is happy with the readings from these monitors, the anaesthetic will start.

The anaesthetist will remain with you throughout the operation to make sure you are asleep and that the function of your heart and lungs is satisfactory. Once the anaesthetic has been injected into the tube in your hand or arm, you will fall asleep within seconds. The drug which makes you go to sleep may sting a little as it enters the vein from the cannula, but this feeling does not last long.

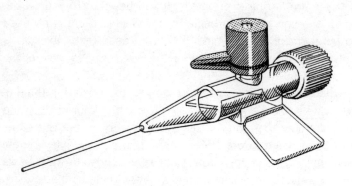

A Butterfly cannula. An example of one type of cannula through which drugs can be injected into a vein (often in the back of the hand) during an operation.

During your operation

Several different types of drugs will be given to you during your operation:

* *induction agents* to bring on sleep;
* *maintenance agents* to keep you asleep;
* *analgesics* to stop you feeling pain during and after the operation;
* *anti-emetics* to help stop you feeling sick after the operation;
* *muscle relaxants* if you are having a radical prostatectomy.

Analgesics and anti-emetics are also given post-operatively as required.

When the operation is over, the anaesthetist will stop giving you the drugs that were keeping you asleep, and you will be taken to a recovery room.

The recovery room

The nurses in the recovery room are specially trained to care for patients coming round from anaesthetics after an operation. You will stay in this room, still watched over by monitoring equipment, until you are fully awake and ready to be returned to your own ward.

If you are in any pain when you wake up, the staff in the recovery room will be able to give you something to relieve it. This can be an injection, either through the cannula which was used to put you to sleep, or into your arm or leg. After transurethral resection, tablets such as paracetamol will probably be enough, although even these are not always necessary.

Back on the ward

Once you are back on your own ward, the anaesthetist may visit you to ensure that you are having adequate pain relief and have no ill-effects from your operation. Do tell the anaesthetist if you have any concerns or questions.

Side-effects of general anaesthesia

There are some side-effects related to the use of general anaesthetics, but these are usually minor and do not last very long. The most common are nausea and vomiting. You may have a sore throat after your operation, possibly due to the 'dry' anaesthetic gases used to keep you asleep during surgery, or to the tube which may have been used to help you to breathe. Whatever the reason, any soreness usually disappears after two or three days and can be eased by the use of simple painkillers.

PAIN RELIEF

The house surgeon and nurses on your ward will be able to give you analgesics if you have any pain. However, if these are not enough, do tell the anaesthetist or ward staff, who may be able to give you something more effective.

The amount of discomfort suffered after any operation varies from person to person, and of course depends on the extent of the surgery involved.

Patient-controlled analgesia

In some hospitals, patient-controlled analgesia (PCA) may be offered after a radical prostatectomy if required, but PCA machines are expensive and may not be available for all patients. The PCA technique has been designed to allow patients themselves to control the amount of analgesic they receive and it is generally a more effective way of providing pain relief than the conventional forms of pain-killing injections.

The machine is basically a pump which delivers a pain-killing drug into your body each time you press a button. It is pro-grammed to allow you only a safe limit of the drug, which is usually delivered via a cannula in a vein in your hand or arm or directly into the skin on your lower abdomen. Once you press the button, your pain should start to reduce within five to ten minutes. If it does not do so, press the button again. As the machine has a built-in safety control to prevent you receiving too much of the drug, you can press the button as often as you like. However, it is important that you do not let anyone else use your machine as this removes the safety feature. If, despite pressing the button several times, your pain is not being relieved, tell a nurse or doctor so that the machine can be reset to deliver a stronger dose of the drug, if this is appropriate.

A nurse or doctor will inspect the counter on your machine every day or so to see how many times you have pressed the button and how much analgesic drug you have received. Once it is clear that you are reducing the amount of drug you need, and therefore your pain is improving, the machine setting will be changed to deliver a lower dose at each press of the button. When patient-controlled analgesia is needed after a radical prostatectomy, it can normally be replaced with analgesic tablets after 24 to 48 hours.

CHAPTER 6

The operations

The type of operation you have will depend largely on the nature of your prostate problem, although the final decision can sometimes only be made once you are anaesthetised and your prostate gland has been examined using a cystoscope (see p.28). You should receive comprehensive counselling before any type of prostate surgery, and be given clear explanations of any possible side-effects you may experience.

TRANSURETHRAL RESECTION OF THE PROSTATE

This operation is done to relieve bladder outflow obstruction secondary to benign prostatic hyperplasia and also sometimes to relieve the symptoms of prostate cancer.

A spinal anaesthetic is usually given, with or without a sedative to put you to sleep, although general anaesthesia is sometimes used. Once the anaesthetic has taken effect, your legs will be put into stirrups to keep them apart (the lithotomy position). Your legs and lower body will then be covered with drapes, and your perineum and genitals cleaned with antiseptic.

A cystoscope will be inserted through your urethra to enable the surgeon to examine the inside of your prostate gland and bladder. A camera is often attached to the cystoscope so that the surgeon can see the operation on a video monitor as he or she performs it.

Your urethra, prostate and bladder will be examined to make sure there is no other cause of your symptoms, such as a

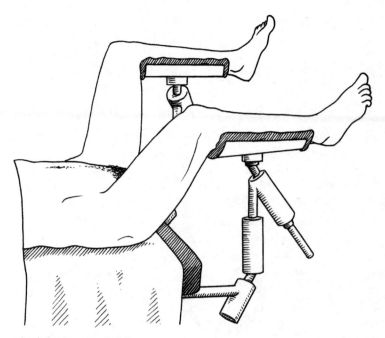

The lithotomy position.

urethral stricture (see p.12) or a bladder stone, and to assess the size of the prostate. A resectoscope (see p.29) will then be introduced into your bladder and an electric current will be passed through the wire loop at its end. The current is used to core out tissue from each half of the prostate gland and from its centre. The pieces of tissue will fall into the bladder and, together with any blood clots, can be washed out using an evacuator. Any little blood vessels which are bleeding will be cauterised at the end of the operation. A plastic catheter will then be passed into your bladder to allow further drainage and irrigation to keep the urine flowing. You may be given a drug after your operation to increase your production of urine and help wash out your bladder.

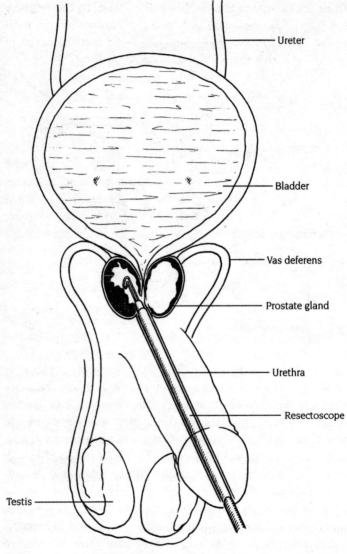

Ureter

Bladder

Vas deferens

Prostate gland

Urethra

Resectoscope

Testis

Transurethral resection of the prostate. The resectoscope is inserted through the urethra and moved to cut away the prostate tissue as shown.

Once the operation is over, you will be taken to the recovery room (see p.53) where you will remain for an hour or so until you have come round from the anaesthetic and the recovery staff are happy that there is no significant bleeding.

BLADDER NECK INCISION

This operation employs basically the same technique as a transurethral resection except that the resectoscope has a single-bladed, knife-like instrument at its end rather than a wire loop. One or two full-length cuts are made in the prostate from the bladder neck downwards so that the prostate tissue which has been pressing on the urethra falls away from it, allowing the urine to flow unobstructed. This operation is only really suitable for small prostates.

OPEN PROSTATECTOMY

An open prostatectomy can be **retropubic** (also known as **Millin's prostatectomy**) or **transvesical**. The prostate itself is opened in the former operation, and the bladder in the latter.

You will be given a spinal or general anaesthetic and an incision will be made in your lower abdominal wall. The peritoneum (the membrane which lines the abdominal and upper pelvic cavities and which encloses the organs within them) is left intact and thus the abdominal cavity is not entered. Either the bladder or the prostate gland will then be opened and the surgeon will use a finger to remove the central part of the prostate. Any bleeding vessels will then be cauterised and a urinary catheter inserted before the hole in the bladder or prostate is stitched. A drain will be put through the body wall, and the incision will be closed with stitches.

You will be taken to the recovery room if you are still asleep, and then back to your ward.

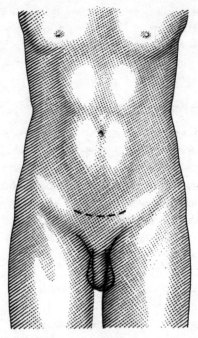

Line of incision for an open prostatectomy.

RADICAL PROSTATECTOMY

This operation involves the complete removal of the prostate gland, the capsule which surrounds it, and both seminal vesicles.

Your bowel may be washed out prior to surgery and you will have been given low-dose heparin injections (see p.43) and antibiotics.

General anaesthesia is commonly used for a radical prostatectomy, although the choice of anaesthetic will depend partly on the normal practice of your particular hospital. An epidural is often inserted for pain relief, and may be left in for several hours post-operatively.

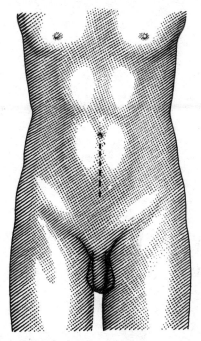

Line of incision for a radical prostatectomy.

Once the anaesthetic has taken effect, you will be laid on your back on the operating table and an incision will be made in your abdominal wall between your navel and pubis. As for an open prostatectomy, the peritoneal membrane will not be cut and your abdominal cavity will not be entered. A catheter will be inserted into your bladder and the entire prostate gland and seminal vesicles will be cut away. When these organs have been removed there will be a gap between your bladder and urethra, which will be closed by stitching the two together with five or six stitches over the catheter, which acts as a splint. One or two wound drains will be inserted and the incision in your abdominal wall will be stitched before you are taken to the recovery room to come round from the anaesthetic.

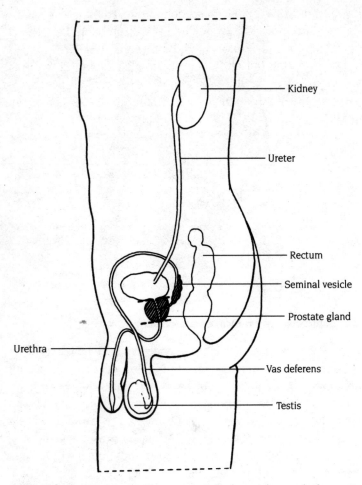

Radical prostatectomy. The two seminal vesicles and the entire prostate gland (shaded) are removed, as well as the section of urethra between the dashed lines.

PELVIC NODE DISSECTION

If you have a pelvic node dissection at the same time as a radical prostatectomy, the lymph nodes will probably be excised first. The group of nodes which drain lymph from the prostate will be dissected out and the lymph vessels tied off. If there is any doubt about whether the lymph nodes contain malignant tissue, they will be sent immediately to the histology laboratory for examination while you are still anaesthetised.

Once the results have been obtained, a decision will be made about whether or not to proceed to radical prostatectomy. If there is already cancer in the pelvic nodes, the prostate gland will not be removed as doing so will not eliminate these regional metastases. Your surgeon should have discussed this possibility with you beforehand. If this happens, the surgeon will explain the findings to you and talk about other treatment options when you are back on your ward.

ORCHIDECTOMY

This operation is now not commonly performed as similar effects can be obtained with hormone injections or tablets. When it is done to treat prostate disease, both testes are removed.

A general anaesthetic is normally given, although local or spinal anaesthesia can be used. A single incision will probably be made across your scrotum and either your testes will be cut away completely or the hormone-producing tissue will be removed from the inside and the lining sewn back together. The incision in the scrotum will then be closed with dissolvable stitches. Wound drains are not usually necessary, but your scrotum is likely to be bruised for a time.

CHAPTER 7

After your operation

What happens after your operation will largely depend on the type of surgery you have had. This chapter gives some idea of what to expect post-operatively, both in hospital and when you are at home again.

IN HOSPITAL

Transurethral surgery to treat benign conditions does not involve abdominal incisions or the post-operative pain associated with them. Therefore the recovery period may be quite short. As the digestive system is not involved in a transurethral resection, you will be able to eat as soon as you want to after your operation. However, recovery takes a little longer following an open or radical prostatectomy: you will have some abdominal pain, and you will not be able to eat for a day or two until you have gradually built up your fluid intake.

After surgery other than a radical prostatectomy

The prostate is a very vascular gland, and after a transurethral resection, open prostatectomy or bladder neck incision there can be quite heavy bleeding. When you return to the ward after surgery, a catheter will be in place to drain urine from your bladder. It will be removed once bleeding has reduced and you will probably be able to pass urine spontaneously after two to three days. Fluid will also be passed through the catheter to break up and remove any clots of blood. A close check will be kept on your fluid balance while you are in hospital to make sure the amount of urine you are passing relates to the amount of fluid you are taking in. Therefore it is important that you always ask a nurse to empty your catheter bag rather than doing it yourself. Once your catheter has been removed, you should urinate into a bottle so that your urine output can continue to be measured.

You will be able to get out of bed the day after your operation. The catheter will be strapped to your leg with the collecting bag attached to a stand so that you can walk around.

You should drink as much as possible (ideally about 3 litres of fluid a day) to help flush the blood from your bladder. Your urine will gradually change from a claret colour, through rose to clear, possibly by the end of the first post-operative day although it may take longer. Once most of the blood has cleared from your urine, you can reduce your daily fluid intake to about 1.5 litres.

After radical prostatectomy

Although you may lose some blood during the operation itself, there is less bleeding after a radical prostatectomy than after most other types of prostate surgery as the entire prostate has been removed.

When you awake after a radical prostatectomy, you will have a urinary catheter, one or two wound drains, and an intravenous drip. The catheter in this case acts as a splint to support the join between the bladder and urethra as it heals. Specially balanced fluids are delivered via the intravenous drip to replace the fluid lost during your operation.

When the amount of blood and fluid leaking from the abdominal wound reduces, probably after a couple of days, the drain(s) will be taken out. You will be given pain relief intravenously, by epidural or by patient-controlled analgesia (see p.54). Your fluid intake will gradually be increased over a couple of days until you are able to eat a light and then a normal diet. You will continue to be given low-dose heparin injections until you are mobile (see p.43).

The intravenous drip will be taken down when you are able to drink again, after which you should try to drink about 2 litres of fluid a day.

You will probably leave hospital within five to seven days after your operation, still with your urinary catheter in place. After a further one or two weeks, you will be asked to return to hospital for a **cystogram**. A cystogram is done by injecting a dye down the side of the urinary catheter and taking a series of X-rays. The X-rays will detect any leaks in the join between your bladder and urethra. If healing is complete, the catheter can then be removed; if not, it will have to remain in place for a further week or two. Once the catheter has been taken out you can start doing pelvic floor exercises to help you regain control of your bladder.

EXERCISES

If you had to strain to pass urine before your operation, it will be a few days before the muscles of your bladder return to a relaxed state. Once the urinary catheter has been removed following any type of prostate surgery, some simple exercises to tighten the perineal muscles around your urethra will help to prevent urine leakage. It is a good idea to practise these exercises before your operation to get used to doing them. The more often you do them post-operatively, the sooner you will regain bladder control.

Exercise 1

Every time you urinate, tighten your perineal muscles by trying to stop the flow of urine for a few seconds midstream.

Exercise 2

Standing upright, pull in your stomach muscles, count to ten, and relax. Do this exercise each time you stand up, and at least every hour to gain maximum effect.

Exercise 3

While standing, sitting or lying down, tighten the muscles of your anus by pulling them up as though you were trying to stop a bowel motion. Do this exercise every ten minutes or so, while breathing normally.

LEAVING HOSPITAL

You will be able to leave hospital after a transurethral resection once you have gained enough control over your bladder. There will probably still be some blood in your urine, causing it to be slightly pink. After a radical prostatectomy, you will go home with the urinary catheter still in place.

It is best to ask someone to collect you from hospital as you should not drive yourself for at least a couple of weeks. If necessary, you may be able to make use of hospital transport, but you should ask a nurse about arranging this in good time if you think you may need it.

When you leave hospital, you may be given a letter to deliver to your doctor's surgery as soon as possible, although it may be sent by post from the hospital.

AT HOME

Once you are at home, you will have to take things easy for a while. Of course, people recover from surgery at different rates but, depending on the type of operation you have had, it may be several weeks at least until you feel any real benefit.

Returning to normal activity

You may feel tired and a bit depressed for anything from a few days to a few weeks. This is quite normal and will eventually pass. You should take things easy for a couple of weeks, going on only short walks (less than a mile) and avoiding driving and any strenuous activity. Sports such as golf and cycling should not be resumed for four to six weeks after a transurethral resection, and for about three months after a radical prostatectomy. You may not feel the full benefits of your operation for several weeks; for some men recovery is not complete for up to six months.

Sexual activity

Until your internal wound has had a chance to heal, sexual intercourse may cause it to bleed and should be avoided for about six weeks.

Fluid intake and urine output

You should continue to drink plenty – about 2 litres a day for the first week you are at home and then as much as possible. However, unless you avoid drinking in the evenings you may need to get up in the night to urinate. You may continue to experience some leakage of urine, and possibly need to urinate frequently and during the night, but these effects will gradually resolve. You can wear a small pad (available from any pharmacy) inside your underpants if urine leaks when you laugh or cough. If you continue to have continence problems, ask at your doctor's surgery to see a district nurse or for a referral to a nurse specialist for advice.

You may pass a small amount of blood through your urethra when you have a bowel motion, but this is normal and nothing to worry about.

Constipation

Constipation can be a problem in the first few days after surgery, and you may be given suppositories while you are in hospital to overcome it. Once you are at home, you should avoid becoming constipated as straining may cause the internal wound to bleed. You may need to take laxatives if a high-fibre diet does not help. Ask your doctor's advice if the problem persists.

Returning to work

Unless you have a heavy manual job, you will probably be able to return to work about a month after most types of prostate surgery, or after two or three months following a radical prosta-tectomy. If you are in any doubt, ask your doctor's advice and for a certificate to enable you to stay off work, which can be renewed on request.

FOLLOW-UP APPOINTMENTS

You will probably have an appointment to see the consultant some time after your operation so that your progress can be checked. Do make a note of any questions you have so that you can ask them at this time.

You may see your consultant for a check-up about six weeks after a transurethral resection or bladder neck incision, by which time the results of the histological examination of the tissue removed from your prostate will be available.

You will probably be seen about three to four weeks after a radical prostatectomy to have a cystogram (see p.66), and again at three months. A blood test will be done at each appointment to measure your PSA level (see p.19). If the prostate gland and cancer have been removed completely, your PSA level should have returned to normal. If all is well, you may be seen again after a further three months, and perhaps six monthly thereafter to check your PSA level and make sure any incontinence or impotence is improving. The intervals between your check-ups will depend on the normal practice of your consultant. Men with advanced prostate cancer are likely to have check-ups every three to six months.

Possible complications of surgery

All operations carry a small risk of general complications such as deep vein thrombosis or chest infection, but there are also other possible complications specifically related to prostate surgery. Although minor post-operative problems are fairly common, serious ones are rare. However, it is as well to be aware of what could go wrong so that you know when to seek medical advice.

GENERAL COMPLICATIONS

Apart from the complications possible after any type of surgery, there are some minor side-effects associated with the use of general anaesthesia, but these should only last a day or two.

Sore throat

You may have a sore throat for a couple of days after a general anaesthetic. This is due to the 'dry' anaesthetic gases or to a tube being put down your throat to help you breathe.

Muscle aches

The muscle relaxants used during anaesthesia can cause muscle aches and pains, but these should pass off within about 48 hours.

71

Chest infection

Chest infection is possible following general anaesthesia for any type of operation. It is particularly common in smokers. Deep breathing is important post-operatively to keep the lungs clear, and if necessary a physiotherapist will visit you on the ward to advise you about appropriate exercises.

Pyrexia

Pyrexia is fever. It can occur in the first 24 hours after surgery but if it persists, its cause will have to be investigated. After prostate surgery it is most likely to indicate a urinary tract infection, although it may be due to a chest or wound infection or to deep vein thrombosis. Urinary infection can occasionally result in **bacteraemia** (bacteria in the circulating blood) or, rarely, **septicaemia** (a more severe infection involving the invasion of the blood by large numbers of bacteria which spread throughout the body). Antibiotics are therefore sometimes given for a few days after surgery to reduce this risk, particularly if a catheter was in place before the operation.

Deep vein thrombosis

Deep vein thrombosis can occur following any type of operation, particularly pelvic surgery (see p.42). Precautions such as the wearing of anti-embolism stockings and a course of low-dose heparin injections while you are in hospital (see p.43) should help to prevent it. It occurs when blood clots form in the deep veins of the body – usually in the calf veins of the legs. Treatment at an early stage can reduce the risk of the blood clot breaking away and lodging, for example, in the lungs, causing a pulmonary embolism, which can have more serious consequences. Thrombosis can be treated with a course of higher-dose heparin injections or long-acting tablets such as warfarin.

AFTER TRANSURETHRAL RESECTION

Serious complications are not common after this type of surgery.

Pain

You are unlikely to experience any severe pain following a transurethral resection of the prostate, and any discomfort you do have should be controlled by simple painkillers such as paracetamol. You should not take aspirin as they have a blood-thinning effect which can increase bleeding. If you have a medical condition for which you normally take aspirin, you will probably have been told not to do so for a few weeks.

Bleeding

Bleeding may occur immediately after surgery and the bladder may be irrigated to remove any clots of blood. Once bleeding has stopped, it is possible for it to start again a week or two later as the scab on the prostate drops off, but this is not a cause for concern and should soon cease if you rest and drink plenty of fluid. Very rarely, bleeding is heavy enough to require re-admission to hospital or even return to the operating theatre.

Transurethral resection syndrome

The fluid used to irrigate the bladder during and immediately after surgery is sometimes absorbed by the body, very rarely resulting in a syndrome due to fluid overload and swelling of tissues, and possibly a confused mental state. If this syndrome occurs, your fluid intake will be reduced and you will be given diuretics to help the body excrete the excess.

Retrograde ejaculation

After transurethral resection or prostatectomy, the bladder muscles are weakened and during ejaculation semen passes backwards into the bladder, sometimes causing the urine to become cloudy. This fairly common condition is known as retrograde ejaculation and is likely to reduce fertility. Althout it is included here for convenience, it is in fact a side-effect rather than a complication. You should therefore discuss this possibility with your doctor before you decide to have an operation if you are planning to have children. However, a prostate operation must not be viewed as a type of contraception as there is no guarantee that you will be sterile after it.

Repeat surgery

Between 1 in 10 and 1 in 20 men will require further prostate surgery during their lives, possibly due to one of three reasons. The prostate may regrow or there may be residual prostate tissue which needs further surgery; scarring can develop in the urethra (a stricture) or bladder neck (bladder neck stenosis) where the prostate has been resected.

AFTER RADICAL (OR OPEN) PROSTATECTOMY

There is inevitably a wider range of complications which can occur after more invasive surgery, and you should ask your doctor's advice if you are at all concerned.

Pain

Although it is normal to have some pain in the abdominal wound after an open or radical prostatectomy, it is unusual for it to be severe. Severe, persistent pain may be a sign that an infection is developing, which will require medical attention (see p.76).

Bleeding and bruising

There is often a certain amount of oozing of blood or fluid from the abdominal wound, but this is unlikely to be heavy. If it continues, and particularly if leakage occurs through the wound dressing and soils your clothes, medical advice should be sought. On rare occasions, a second operation is required to tie off or cauterise a bleeding blood vessel which was overlooked or which started to bleed again post-operatively.

Occasionally, blood which does not escape through the edges of the wound may lead to severe bruising, sometimes developing several days after surgery. Although the sight of the bruise may be distressing, treatment is only seldom required to release the blood which has accumulated under the skin.

Haematoma

In rare cases, a haematoma may develop. A haematoma is a collection of blood, and is a complication which can occur after any type of operation. The swelling can vary in size, and is caused by a blood vessel continuing to bleed or re-bleeding after surgery. People taking anticoagulants are more likely to bleed. There are also inherited bleeding disorders, such as haemophilia, which cause a similar disturbance of the blood-clotting mechanism, but these conditions will be taken into account before any operation is considered.

Haematoma development may be accompanied by pain and the formation of a swelling if it is close to the skin surface, and possibly a reddish purple discoloration of the skin. Bruising may appear around the wound or at some distance from it over the next few days. A raised body temperature may develop if the haematoma becomes infected.

If you think a haematoma is forming or has formed once you have left hospital, you should contact your family doctor or consultant for advice. The blood is likely to be reabsorbed spontaneously within three or four weeks without the need for any treatment, but sometimes it has to be drained out. Rarely, if heavy bleeding continues, with increased pain and swelling, you may need surgery to close off the blood vessel which is causing it. Your doctor may also wish to do specialised blood tests to check that your blood-clotting factors are normal.

Wound infection

Infection can sometimes occur in the abdominal wound following a prostatectomy and is indicated by pain, swelling, heat and redness around the wound, possibly with leakage of pus or infected fluid and a high body temperature. As most modern wound dressings are transparent, it is now much easier to examine wounds for signs of infection.

If an infection develops, it may be enough simply for the wound to be cleansed, or it may require treatment with antibiotics. Occasionally, some of the stitches, which provide potential sites for the concentration of germs, may have to be removed to allow an infected discharge to escape. You should seek medical attention if you have any signs of an infection.

Very occasionally, possibly weeks or months after surgery, infection can arise from suture materials that have been left within the wound.

Nerve damage

Small nerves supplying the skin over the lower abdomen are frequently cut when an incision is made during surgery, causing a small area around the wound to remain permanently numb. Although the size of the area of numbness will decrease with time, the sensation may never return completely.

Very rarely, small, painful, tender areas form in part of the scar, which may be due to a swelling of the cut nerve ends known as a **neuroma**. Nerve damage may lead to pain in the wound which will be relieved temporarily by the injection of local anaesthetic. Continued pain may respond to steroid injection. Only rarely is surgery needed to remove a painful nodule.

Constipation

Constipation is common in the first few days after any operation. You may be given laxative suppositories while in hospital to avoid straining to empty your bowel. You should have a high-fibre diet once you are at home but if constipation persists, ask your doctor's advice about taking a laxative.

Difficulty in passing urine

Passing urine may be difficult for several days after a prostatectomy, sometimes due to pain, infection or a blood clot. If urinary retention occurs, a catheter may have to be left in place longer to empty the bladder until you are able to urinate spontaneously. Always seek medical advice if you appear to be retaining urine.

Leakage of urine

Although the leakage of urine caused by an enlarged prostate usually improves following surgery, it can get worse in the immediate post-operative period while the bladder muscles regain their tone.

It is also possible for the operation itself to affect the sphincter which closes off the flow of urine from the bladder. This is likely to be only a temporary effect which will improve with time.

Stenosis

Occasionally, urine comes out in a spray or narrow stream after surgery due to constriction (stenosis or stricture) of the neck of the bladder. If necessary, this can be corrected by a small operation to dilate the bladder neck.

Incontinence

Temporary incontinence is relatively common after radical prostate surgery and may persist for weeks or even months. However, some 3 to 5 per cent of prostate operations result in permanent incontinence which may require an operation to insert an artificial urinary sphincter.

Reduced fertility

Fertility may be reduced after an open prostatectomy due to retrograde ejaculation (see p.74). Semen is no longer produced after a radical prostatectomy and men who have had this operation are therefore rendered sterile.

Loss of libido

A loss of interest in sex occasionally follows the removal of the prostate gland and this is a possibility you should consider and discuss with your doctor before your operation. To some men, loss of libido is not of great concern, particularly to those whose symptoms were affecting their day-to-day life, but others are anxious about this risk.

Impotence

Impotence is relatively common following radical prostate surgery and should be discussed with your surgeon before your operation.

Other sexual effects

A significant proportion of men experience a change in their sensation of orgasm after prostate surgery, which for some reduces their enjoyment of sex. Some men find it more difficult to get an erection, although this can result from any type of surgery, not just from a prostate operation.

RISKS OF GENERAL ANAESTHESIA

The use of a general anaesthetic always involves a certain risk. Although the advances in anaesthesia over the past few years have been tremendous, complications still occur and, on very rare occasions, people do die during routine operations. Therefore, the small but real risks need to be understood and considered.

If circulatory problems interrupt the supply of oxygen to the brain during anaesthesia, there are two possible outcomes: death may occur without the patient ever waking up; or the patient may wake brain damaged and possibly paralysed. However, these risks are small, and careful consideration will have been given by the surgeon and the anaesthetist to your general state of health and all other relevant factors before deciding to go ahead with your operation and anaesthesia.

CHAPTER 9

Radiotherapy

This chapter gives a general description of how radiotherapy is given as a primary treatment for prostate cancer (instead of surgery). Some of the details are the same when it is used to relieve symptoms of bone pain in advanced disease, but specific aspects of palliative treatment are dealt with on p.87.

Radiotherapy is sometimes the treatment of choice for younger men with localised disease or with local spread around the prostate gland. It involves the use of high-energy radiation (X-rays) to destroy cancer cells. Although the X-rays damage the DNA in all cells in the targeted area, normal cells can usually repair themselves within a couple of hours, whereas the cancer cells take longer to do so and, after repeated radiation treatment, are eventually relatively selectively destroyed. If there is suspicion that the cancer has spread to the regional pelvic lymph nodes, these may also sometimes be treated with radiotherapy.

RECEIVING YOUR TREATMENT

Radiotherapy as a primary treatment is usually given in several separate sessions, possibly every weekday for six weeks or more, each lasting only a few minutes. Before the treatment starts, a total radiation dose is calculated and divided into several smaller amounts to be given at each treatment session. Although different treatment centres may divide the total dose differently, the outcome is generally the same.

* **Radiologists** are doctors trained to interpret X-rays and in the administration of dyes etc. which are used for some types of X-ray examination.
* **Radiographers** are technicians who have undergone a three-year degree course and are qualified to operate X-ray machinery and to administer radiation treatment under the guidance of a doctor.
* **Radiotherapists** (or **radiation oncologists**) are doctors who specialise in the treatment of cancer using radiation. Most also administer other types of cancer treatment, such as chemotherapy.
* **Oncologists** are physicians who have specialist training in all aspects of cancer, particularly radiotherapy and chemotherapy, but not surgery.

If you are to have radiotherapy, you may be sent an appointment for pre-teatment planning so that the doctor can decide how best to administer it. The doctor in charge of your treatment may be a clinical oncologist or a radiotherapist (see above). During the pre-treatment planning or on your first visit for radiotherapy, a radiographer will explain the procedures to you. Do ask any questions, however trivial they may seem, and do not be afraid to ask for something to be explained again if you have not understood it. If you are at all worried as your treatment progresses, talk to the radiographer again on a subsequent visit.

When you enter the treatment room for your first radiotherapy session, you will be asked to lie on a couch and the doctor will mark out on your skin with a felt-tip pen the area to be treated. The X-ray machine will be lowered until it almost touches your abdomen. You will be told to keep very still while treatment is in progress.

Once the machine has been set up, all the medical staff will leave the treatment room to protect themselves against repeated exposure to radiation. A radiographer will watch you closely through a window or on a television monitor. If you are concerned or require any assistance, simply raise your hand and the process will be stopped immediately. There will also be an intercom system so the radiographer can hear and speak to you. The treatment only lasts a couple of minutes.

> **Hostel wards** Some hospitals have hostel wards, usually open from Monday to Friday, for use by people who would have to travel some distance each day for their treatment. The hostel wards provide a bed and meals and although they are not staffed by nurses, there is always someone in charge of them. These wards are suitable for people who are able to look after themselves, and are therefore ideal for those undergoing daily radiotherapy treatment who are otherwise in good health.
>
> Do ask your doctor before your treatment starts about the availability of hostel ward beds if appropriate.

SIDE-EFFECTS

Some men experience side-effects which usually cease with the end of their radiation treatment. Others suffer no ill-effects and are able to continue their normal activities between treatment sessions. If you do feel tired during and immediately after your course of treatment, it may be sensible to arrange to work part-time while it lasts so that you can rest when you need to.

Diarrhoea, cystitis-like problems and the passage of blood in the urine are not uncommon during radiotherapy as parts of the bowel and the bladder are included in the treatment area. The side-effects can be quite severe and a small number of men are left with more permanent problems. Tell the radiographer or a doctor if you experience side-effects as there are medicines to help relieve diarrhoea and ways to manage frequent micturition.

You will lose any hair within the treated area, but it will regrow once treatment stops.

There is a 30 to 40 per cent risk of impotence following radical radiotherapy, and this possibility should be explained and discussed with you before your treatment starts.

CHAPTER 10

Treatment of advanced prostate cancer

Radiotherapy or hormone therapy may slow the growth of advanced prostate cancer or help relieve its symptoms. These treatments, which may sometimes prevent a prostate cancer from growing for many months or years but which cannot cure it, are called **palliative**. Chemotherapy is rarely used to treat prostate cancer. Although it is sometimes a palliative treatment for other types of metastatic cancer, it is relatively ineffective for prostate cancer.

For people whose cancer is incurable, there is now a good deal of care and support available from hospices and specially trained nurses based in hospitals, cancer centres and the community, and much that can be done to make living with cancer a less frightening and stressful experience for sufferers and their families. Palliative care is not just for people who are about to die; it is long-term care that can continue for months or years, and many take advantage of the support that is available to improve their quality of life.

In Britain, hospice-based care and the support of Macmillan nurses (see p.89) are free to all who need them, and are funded by charities or by the National Health Service.

HORMONE THERAPY

Hormone therapy makes use of the various hormones produced by the body which affect the growth and function of its organs. It can be used to shrink a prostate cancer or to slow its rate of growth by removing the testosterone drive to the cancer cells (and to the benign cells). However, there is no firm evidence that *early* hormone treatment improves the survival of men with prostate cancer. Of those who already have metastatic disease in the bones when hormone treatment is started, 60 to 70 per cent respond well, 10 to 20 per cent respond reasonably, and 10 to 20 per cent show no response.

There are various types of hormone therapy, the clinical effects of which are probably identical.

Bilateral orchidectomy

The main male hormone involved in prostate cancer is testosterone, produced by the testes. Bilateral orchidectomy (see p.63), although a surgical procedure to remove both testes, is strictly a hormone treatment in that it results in the loss of the main source of testosterone.

LHRH analogues

Production of testosterone is under the control of another hormone called luteinising hormone (LH) which is produced by the pituitary gland in the brain. This in turn is controlled by luteinising hormone-releasing hormone (LHRH), produced in the hypothalamus in the brain. Various drugs have been developed to treat prostate cancer which are artificial forms of LHRH (analogues) and which, if given over a long period of time, stop the pituitary gland producing LH and thus prevent the production of testosterone.

The LHRH analogues are usually given as injections, either once every 4 weeks or once every 12 weeks. The most commonly used form in the UK is Zoladex (goserelin), but others are used in different countries, for example Prostap and Decapeptyl.

Zoladex is a pellet which is injected under the skin of the abdominal wall, with our without the use of a local anaesthetic. Other forms of the drug are injected intramuscularly into the buttock or leg. The first injection may be given by your consultant, or sometimes by a radiotherapist or oncologist, but subsequent injections are often given by family doctors.

There is an initial complication with the use of the LHRH analogues in that they tend to turn the regulatory system of the pituitary *up* for a couple of weeks, thus increasing the levels of hormone produced in the body. This effect is reduced by giving the drugs in combination with an anti-androgen called cyproterone acetate (see below) for the first couple of weeks until the hormone system has turned itself off.

Anti-androgens

Androgens are male steroid hormones, the commonest of which is testosterone, produced in the testes. Other androgens produced by the adrenal glands also appear to be involved in controlling prostate cancers, although there is debate about their degree of importance. Anti-androgens are another group of drugs used to treat prostate cancer. They include flutamide, casodex and a slightly different drug called cyproterone acetate (which is also sometimes used to reduce the libido of male sex offenders). They are given as tablets, sometimes for many years. The drugs block the effect of the male hormones on prostate cancer cells; cyproterone acetate also affects the production of male hormones by the brain. Some urologists feel that anti-androgens alone are less effective than other drugs in controlling the male hormonal drive to prostate cancer cells, and prefer LHRH analogues. However, cyproterone acetate is still often used as a first-line treatment. The anti-androgens do have side-effects. Flutamide and casodex can cause breast pain, breast enlargement and gastrointestinal problems; cyproterone acetate may induce shortness of breath and tiredness.

Maximal androgen blockade

Another form of hormone therapy is maximal androgen blockade, which combines orchidectomy *or* the use of LHRH analogues with anti-androgens. It has been suggested that this treatment may improve the survival for younger men (in their fifties and sixties) with advanced disease, but it is not in general use in Britain at the present time.

Oestrogens

In the past, a group of female hormones called oestrogens were used to treat advanced prostate cancer. Although these were effective in controlling the cancer, they had a higher level of side-effects than the other treatments mentioned here. At high doses, they tend to cause feminisation, including enlargement of the breasts and breast pain, and increase the risk of heart disease when taken in the long term. They are therefore not now used routinely.

RADIOTHERAPY

Apart from its use as a curative treatment for localised prostate cancer in younger men (see Chapter 9), radiotherapy can be a useful treatment to relieve bone pain in men with advanced disease. It may be given at the same time as hormone therapy or afterwards if hormone therapy becomes ineffective. A single treatment of the affected area is sometimes enough to relieve bone pain, but it will take seven to ten days for its effects to become fully apparent. Alternatively, the radiation dose can be divided into fractions given at several treatment sessions over a week or two.

For severe bone pain due to multiple, widespread metastases, a single high dose of radiation may be given to half the body (**hemi-body radiotherapy**). Alternatively, a radioactive liquid (strontium-89) may be injected into a vein. Strontium-89 is taken up by the areas of bone affected by the cancer and the radiation is released inside the bone itself. This treatment does not become fully effective for about three or four weeks. It is quite successful at relieving bone pain and it can be repeated after three or four months. The bone marrow may be affected, causing anaemia, susceptibility to infection and bleeding disorders.

Prostate cancer in the advanced stages can affect the bones of the spine, sometimes putting pressure on the nerves of the spinal cord. This is a serious condition which can lead to permanent paralysis unless it is treated promptly with radiotherapy. Therefore, if you develop weakness of the legs or numbness of the skin, you should report these symptoms to your doctor immediately.

HOSPICES

For men with metastatic prostate cancer which cannot be cured, hospice involvement may be suggested by their family doctor, consultant or a specialist cancer nurse. Many people are shocked at this suggestion as they imagine hospices to be places to go to die. But although some people choose to spend their last days in a hospice, their main role is to support cancer patients, and their families, and to help them remain well and to live as full and normal a life as possible for as long as possible – which in many cases means continuing support for years. Hospice staff work with family doctors to plan the best care for their patients.

Hospices have several aims:

* to help cancer patients live full and happy lives,
* to provide pain relief and to control any other symptoms of cancer which may arise,
* to counsel and support cancer patients and their families,

* to offer advice and information about grants and financial assistance which may be available,
* to provide education and courses on palliative care for nurses and doctors,
* to provide regular home visits to support and care for cancer patients and their families and enable people to be cared for in their own homes rather than in hospitals.

Some hospices also have in-patient facilities where people can go if they have symptoms which need to be brought under control, or simply to give their carers at home a week or two's respite. Many also have day-care facilities where cancer sufferers can spend the day involved in leisure activities such as painting, woodwork or making jewellery, and where they can have their hair done, be bathed if this is becoming difficult at home, talk to a doctor or social worker, or just sit and chat in a friendly and supportive environment.

Specialist nurses based within hospices or in the community work closely with family doctors – who remain in overall charge of their patients' care – as well as with community nurses and social workers. Their special skills and experience enable them to co-ordinate the care their patients receive and to make sure they have the emotional support and medical treatment they require.

Some people prefer not to be referred to a hospice, and some manage well alone. But many who do accept this help find their quality of life and ability to cope with their disease much improved.

MACMILLAN NURSES

The Cancer Relief Macmillan Fund (CRMF) was set up in Britain in 1911 to provide care and support for cancer patients. This national charity now helps to improve the quality of life for cancer patients and their families at home, in hospitals and in special cancer units.

The CRMF has trained over a thousand Macmillan nurses who work in the community and in hospitals around Britain. It continues to fund these specially trained nurses for up to three years in posts in hospitals, after which the health authority takes over the financial responsibility.

A doctor or district nurse may suggest involving a Macmillan nurse to help care for someone with incurable prostate cancer. Macmillan nurses play a similar role to that of hospice-based nurses, giving advice and emotional support to people and their families, and working closely with other medical professionals to advise about pain relief and symptom control as necessary. They are also involved in the training of doctors and nurses to help them develop the special skills required for the care of cancer patients and, with hospice staff, have been largely responsible for the increased awareness of other health professionals to the particular care these patients need.

OTHER TREATMENT CENTRES

The effects of complementary or alternative therapies are difficult to assess, in part because they are often only resorted to by people for whom conventional medicine has no more to offer in terms of cure.

There are a few private centres in the UK which advocate special non-medical therapies to help people 'fight' or live with cancer. Your family doctor, consultant or a specialist nurse should be able to give you details of any such centres in your area, or you can contact one of the associations whose addresses are given in Appendix IV. Alternative therapy centres are not funded by the NHS; some have trust funds to help meet the costs for those who cannot afford them.

CHAPTER 11

Private care

In countries such as Britain where there is a state health service, there are various reasons why people choose to have their operations done privately. They may have private health insurance, or be covered by a private health scheme run by the company for which they work, or they may be able to pay for private care themselves. Whatever your situation, you will not find that the *standard* of medical care you receive in a private hospital is any different from that available on the National Health Service. But you may prefer the privacy of a private hospital, or you may find the opportunity to enter hospital for your operation at the time of your choice is more convenient for you.

If you have an operation in an NHS hospital, you may not see the consultant at all, being examined and treated by different doctors in the consultant's firm. At a private hospital, you will receive personal care from the consultant throughout your stay. The facilities at a private hospital are likely to be similar to those of a good hotel, and will certainly include a private bathroom.

The information given in other chapters in this book is equally relevant whichever system you choose. This chapter explains the practicalities of obtaining private health care and deals with the differences between the two systems.

PRIVATE HEALTH INSURANCE

If you work for a company which has a private health insurance scheme, your Company Secretary will be able to give you details, and should be able to tell you if the company insurance covers you for your operation.

If you have your own private health insurance, someone at the insurance company will be able to tell you exactly what is covered by your particular policy if this is not clear from the literature you already have. It is always worth checking anyway, and asking for *written* confirmation. Do not be afraid to keep asking questions until you are certain you know exactly which costs you will be responsible for paying yourself. For example, does your insurance cover all follow-up appointments?

There are different levels of health insurance, and you need to make sure you know which costs are included. Most private hospitals have an administration officer who will check your policy for you if you are in any doubt. The staff at the hospital are likely to be very helpful and will try to sort out any problems and queries you have. But do read your policy carefully, and any information sent to you by the hospital, as unexpected charges, such as consultants' fees which may not be covered, could add up to quite a lot of money.

With some types of private health insurance, you will need to ask your family doctor to fill in a form stating that your operation is necessary and cannot be done in an NHS hospital within a certain time period due to long waiting lists. You will have to pay your doctor for this service, which will cost a few pounds. This money is not redeemable from your insurers.

FIXED PRICE CARE

If you think you may be able to pay to have your operation done privately, the Bookings Manager at a private hospital can give you an idea of the cost involved. Some private hospitals run a service known as Fixed Price Care: a price can be quoted to you before you enter hospital which covers your operation and a variety of other hospitalisation costs. You should always ask to have the quotation in writing *before* you enter hospital, with a written note of everything it includes. At some hospitals, the fixed price will include accommodation, nursing, meals, drugs, dressings, operating theatre fees, X-rays etc.; at others only some of these are included. Once you have a quotation, you should not have to worry about any hidden costs for which you had not accounted. However, the price quoted to you may not include the fees of the consultant surgeon or anaesthetist, and you may have to ask your consultant for a note of these.

With Fixed Price Care, all the hospitalisation costs included by that particular hospital are covered should a complication arise which is directly related to your prostate problem or the surgery to treat it and which necessitates you staying longer in hospital, usually up to a maximum of 28 days. Again, consultants' fees will probably be extra. However, if you develop some problem while in hospital which is unrelated to your original prostate problem, the price you have been quoted will not cover treatment to deal with this. At some hospitals, the quoted price will also include your treatment should you have to be re-admitted due to a complication related to your original operation and arising within a limited period of time after your discharge.

The only extra charges you will have to pay to the hospital will probably include those for telephone calls, any alcohol if you have this with your meals, food provided for your visitors, personal laundry done by the hospital and any similar items such as you would have to pay for in a hotel. It is usually possible for a visitor to eat meals with you in your room, and for tea and snacks to be ordered for visitors during the day. (You will also have to pay these extra charges before you leave the hospital if you are being treated under private health insurance.)

It is important therefore that you ask in advance for *written confirmation* of the price you will have to pay for your stay in hospital and what is included in the quotation. If the hospital does not have a Fixed Price Care or similar system, make sure that all possible costs are listed.

ARRANGING THE OPERATION

As for treatment under the NHS, you will have to be referred to see a consultant privately by your family doctor. Most doctors have contacts with particular consultants (and private hospitals) to whom they tend to refer patients. If there is a private hospital you particularly want to go to, or a consultant you have some reason to prefer, you can ask your family doctor to make an appointment for you.

After your visit to your doctor, you are unlikely to have to wait longer than a week or two before you see the consultant at an out-patient appointment. Your appointment may be at the private hospital where your operation is to be carried out, at an NHS hospital which has private wards, or at the consultant's private consulting rooms. Once the decision has been made to go ahead with surgery, you will probably be able to enter hospital at your convenience within another week or two.

You will receive confirmation of the date of your operation from the Bookings Manager of the hospital you are to attend. You may also be sent leaflets and any further relevant details about your admission to hospital. Do read these carefully, as knowing how a particular hospital organises things will help you to be prepared when you arrive for your operation. You will also be sent a **pre-admission form** to fill in and take with you when you are admitted.

If your operation is being paid for by insurance, you will be asked to take a completed insurance form with you when you are admitted to hospital. You should have been given some of these forms when you first took out your policy, but your insurance company will be able to supply the correct one if you have any problems. If you are covered by company insurance, the form will probably be filled in and given to you by your Company Secretary.

ADMISSION AND DISCHARGE

When you arrive at the hospital, the receptionist will contact the admissions department, and a ward receptionist will come to collect you. If you are paying for your treatment yourself, you will probably be asked to pay your bill in advance at this stage if you have not already done so. Otherwise, you will be asked for your completed insurance form. The ward receptionist will take you to your room – probably a single or double room – and show you the facilities available there. You are likely to have a private bathroom, a television, and a telephone by your bed. The ward receptionist will explain hospital procedures to you, and will leave you to settle in.

A member of the nursing staff will then come to make a note of your medical details, in much the same way as described in Chapter 4. The main difference you are likely to notice if you have been treated in an NHS hospital before, is that this time there is much less waiting for all the routine hospital procedures to be dealt with. The nurse to patient ratio is higher in private hospitals and so someone is usually available to deal with the pre-operative procedures quite quickly.

Your consultant will take charge of your medical care throughout your stay, will visit you before the operation, perform the operation (with the assistance of the anaesthetist and the operating staff), and visit you again when you are back in your own room. Trainees – whether doctors or nurses – do not work in private hospitals. The consultants are responsible for their own patients and supervise their care themselves. Most private hospitals now have resident medical officers – fully qualified, registered doctors who are available 24 hours a day to deal with any emergencies which may arise.

When the time for your operation approaches, a porter and nurse will take you from your room to the anaesthetic room. In many private hospitals, you will not be moved from your bed onto a trolley until you have been anaesthetised; the bed itself will be wheeled from your room. Similarly, you will be transferred back from the trolley to your own bed in the recovery room while you are still asleep. You therefore go to sleep and wake up in your own hospital bed.

Your operation will be performed in the same way as described in Chapter 6. When you are fully awake, you will be taken back to your room to rest.

When you are ready to be discharged from hospital, the ward receptionist will ask you to pay any outstanding charges not covered by the hospitalisation charge, and you will be given any medical items you may need from the hospital pharmacy.

SUMMARY

The main aim of the staff of any private hospital is the same as that in an NHS hospital – to make your stay as pleasant and as comfortable as possible. Because the staffing ratio is higher in private hospitals, more emphasis can be placed on privacy and comfort.

The consultant surgeons and anaesthetists almost always work in an NHS hospital as well as in a private hospital, so you will receive the same expertise and skill under both systems. However, in an NHS hospital you may not actually be operated on by the consultant surgeon who heads the surgical team and, indeed, you may not see the consultant at all during your stay.

Private hospitals arrange their operating lists differently from NHS hospitals. The latter have 'sessional bookings' for their operating theatres. This means a particular day is set aside at regular intervals for a specialist in one type of surgery to perform operations. In private hospitals, the consultants can book the use of an operating theatre (and the assistance of the staff who work in it) on more or less any day, at any time that suits them. Therefore, your operation can take place privately at a time that is convenient to you and your consultant.

It is also possible, even if you are already on an NHS waiting list, to tell your family doctor or consultant at any time that you would like to change to private care. If the consultant you have already seen under the NHS does not have a private practice, you can ask to be put in touch with one who *can* see you privately.

There are several reasons why, if they can, some people choose to have their operations done privately, either paid for by private health insurance or from their own pockets. Some find it more convenient to be able to have a say in when their operation is to take place. Some simply prefer the smaller, more intimate setting they are likely to find in a private hospital. As private hospitals rarely deal with accidents and emergency treatment (the operations carried out in them normally being planned at least a day or two in advance), they do not have the bustle of an NHS hospital which has to deal with emergency admissions as well as the routine admissions for non-emergency operations.

Questions and answers

1. I have recently started to have to get up three or four times a night to pass water. I also often need to urinate urgently during the day but find it difficult to do so once I get to the toilet, particularly at night. Is it just my age – I am 68 – and something I will have to put up with, or should I go to my doctor?

Your problems may be related to enlargement of your prostate gland, which is age related but not something you have to put up with. However, there could be other causes and you should certainly see your doctor, who will probably refer you to a urology clinic for tests. Treatment will depend on the diagnosis, but you may need surgery to cut back your prostate gland and relieve your symptoms. If possible, make a note over the next few days of how often you urinate and any difficulties you have in passing urine and take it with you when you see your doctor.

2. I am finding it increasingly difficult to urinate: even when my bladder feels full, the urine comes out in a slow trickle, despite straining, and the feeling of fullness never really goes away. I am 52 and otherwise in good health. What could be the cause?

It is normal for the prostate gland to enlarge as you get older, and it can cause obstruction of the urethra, through which urine empties from the bladder. However, symptoms of urinary obstruction can also be caused by urethral stricture and investigations will need to be done. Depending on their findings, a doctor at the urology clinic will explain the treatment options to you.

3. I am 68 and am having difficulty passing urine which I suspect may be due to an enlarged prostate. (My brother recently had surgery for similar problems.) I have not been to my doctor as I do not want to have an operation. Is there an alternative to surgery?

You should see your doctor and have some tests to investigate the cause of your problem. If your prostate is enlarged, an alternative to surgery may be appropriate, such as drug therapy. However, many prostate operations are done by transurethral resection which, unlike open surgery, does not involve making an incision in the abdominal wall. There are also alternatives to general anaesthesia such as a spinal anaesthetic. In any event, the final decision about treatment is yours and you should talk to your doctor about the options and about the specific aspects of surgery which concern you.

4. For the last couple of days I have found it increasingly difficult to pass any urine, despite feeling the need to do so. Is this a temporary problem which will cure itself?

Your problem may resolve spontaneously, but it could be a sign that you are starting to retain urine. Although chronic urinary retention is not particularly painful, it can occasionally lead to kidney damage. Consult your doctor as you may need to have a catheter inserted to drain your bladder and to be examined at a urology clinic to discover the cause of your problem.

5. I am due to have prostate surgery but have been told I may have to wait at least six months. Is it too late to try to find out about having my operation done privately and, if not, who should I ask about the costs involved?

Tell your family doctor that you would like to see a private consultant. If the consultant you have already seen does not have a private practice, your doctor will be able to refer you to one who does. You should be able to remain on the NHS waiting list until you have made a final decision to have your operation done privately. The consultant will be able to give you an idea of the costs involved, but you should also obtain a written estimate of costs from the private hospital before committing yourself to private treatment – it is likely to amount to a quite considerable sum.

6.   *I have been told I have prostate cancer and am due to start radiotherapy next month. Will this cure it, and is it safe to delay starting treatment this long?*

If the cancer is still localised, there is a good chance that radiotherapy will cure it. Prostate cancers are usually slow growing, progressing over a matter of years, so there should be no reason why delaying your treatment for a few weeks will affect your chances of cure. Do talk to your doctor, or ask for an appointment with a nurse specialist at your hospital who can explain your condition and treatment to you.

7.   *My father is waiting to have a radical prostatectomy. My mother is more or less dependent on his care, but will not agree to stay with me while he is in hospital as I live too far away for her to be able to visit him. They are very independent, but I really don't think she will be able to manage alone. Is there anything I can do to make it possible for her to stay in her own home so she can visit my father in hospital each day?*

Contact your parents' local social services department and explain the situation. It should be possible for 'meals on wheels' and a home help to be organised for your mother for as long as necessary, and for your father too once he is home after his operation. Make sure you have first worked out exactly how much and what type of help your mother would need and that you explain her requirements clearly so that suitable arrangements can be made.

8.   Six weeks ago I had an operation to reduce the size of my prostate, but I still have almost the same problems as before – needing to go to the toilet frequently both day and night and tending to leak urine before and after I urinate. Has the operation failed?

It can take several weeks or even months before the effects of prostate surgery become fully apparent, but your problems should gradually improve. The bladder muscles have to regain their tone, and the operation itself can cause bruising and trauma to the urinary system. You can buy pads at any pharmacy to wear in your underpants to absorb any unavoidable urine leaks until this problem resolves. A district nurse or a continence nurse at your hospital will be able to advise you about anything else you can do to improve things. The pelvic floor exercises which you should have been told about while in hospital will also help you regain bladder control. However, incontinence after prostate surgery can occasionally be permanent and if your problems persist, ask your doctor's advice as investigations may be necessary to discover their cause.

9.   I am waiting to have surgery for an enlarged prostate but have recently begun to find passing urine painful and accompanied by a severe burning sensation in my penis. Should I go back to my doctor or just wait until my operation in five weeks time?

It is important to tell your doctor of any change in your symptoms. You may have a urinary infection, which will need to be treated with antibiotics, or you may be starting to retain urine and may need a catheter inserted to drain your bladder.

10.   I have heard that prostate surgery makes men impotent. I am 63 and have been advised that I need a prostatectomy but do not want to have it if this is the case. Is there an alternative with less drastic effects?

There is a risk of some degree of impotency following prostate surgery, estimated at between 10 and 30 per cent, and you should discuss this with your urology consultant. Ask your family doctor to request an appointment for you, or ring the consultant's secretary. Depending on the prostate problem you have, and whether there is any risk to your health if you do not have an operation, it may be possible to reduce your symptoms by other means, such as with drugs. You could ask to talk to a nurse specialist at the hospital who will be able to discuss things with you in more detail.

11.   *I am due to have a prostate operation which I understand will involve open surgery and quite a long scar. A friend had a similar operation but he has no scar at all. Should I find another surgeon who can do it the same way?*

Although most prostate operations are now done through the urethra by inserting instruments into the penis, open prostate surgery is usually necessary to cut back tissue from a very large prostate gland or to remove the prostate altogether, for example for prostate cancer. It sounds as though an open operation is needed in your case, but do ask your family doctor or consultant why this type of surgery has been chosen for you.

12.   *My father is 74 and has various urinary problems which have recently been diagnosed as due to prostate cancer. His doctor has suggested 'watchful waiting' but surely he needs urgent treatment now to get rid of the cancer before it spreads?*

Your father's doctor may feel that an operation is not necessary at the present time if the cancer is small and the symptoms are not severe. If your father's general health is poor and the cancer is likely to grow so slowly as to cause no serious problems during his lifetime, the risks of surgery may be thought to be greater than those posed by the cancer. If the cancer has already spread to other parts of his body, removal of the prostate gland will not cure it, but watchful waiting will enable any further symptoms to be dealt with as they arise.

Your father's situation will be monitored regularly and any action taken as and when it becomes necessary. He should let his doctor know immediately if he detects any change in his symptoms. Do ask to talk to your father's doctor if you are concerned.

13.   I have been told I will probably have to stay in hospital for up to seven days after my prostate operation, but know someone who was discharged after only three days following the same sort of surgery. Why has such a long stay been anticipated for me?

Recovery from a transurethral resection of the prostate, which is done through the urethra and therefore does not necessitate making an incision in the abdominal wall, is usually relatively quick. After an open or radical prostatectomy, on the other hand, for which an abdominal incision is needed, the bladder and bowel take longer to return to normal function as they are handled during surgery. The abdominal wound also needs time to heal. It sounds as though your friend had a transurethral resection and that you require open surgery for a larger prostate or prostate cancer. Do ask you doctor, consultant or a nurse specialist at the hospital to explain things to you.

14.   I am due to have surgery to remove part of an enlarged prostate and have been told it may affect my fertility. Does this mean that my wife and I can stop using contraception?

Following some types of prostate surgery, there is a tendency for semen to pass back into the bladder on ejaculation. Although this is not harmful, it does lead to reduced fertility, but not necessarily to sterility. It would still be possible for some semen and sperm to be ejaculated during sexual intercourse and you and your wife should therefore continue to take contraceptive precautions.

15. *I have been diagnosed as having prostate cancer. What are the chances of it spreading?*

Most cancers will eventually spread to other parts of the body, but the majority of prostate cancers are relatively slow growing, progressing over many years. Depending on your age, you may therefore never suffer any serious symptoms because of it. Treatment before spread has occurred is often effective and your consultant should be able to advise you about the prognosis in your case.

16. *I am due to have a transurethral resection of the prostate. How long will it be before I can go back to work and start playing tennis again?*

Transurethral resection is the least invasive of the prostate operations. It does not involve making an incision in the abdominal wall and recovery usually occurs reasonably quickly. However, the cut surface of the prostate gland itself needs time to heal, and there will inevitably be some minor damage caused to the urethra during surgery.

Everyone recovers at a different rate, and you may feel much as normal after only a few days, although you will probably continue to feel quite tired and need to take things easy for about two weeks at least. You should avoid driving during this period and should not play tennis or undertake any other strenuous activities for four to six weeks. Unless you do heavy manual work, you may feel able to return to it within two to four weeks post-operatively, but your family doctor should be able to advise you about this.

17. *I have been diagnosed as having prostate cancer. Could my wife catch it through sexual intercourse with me?*

No. Women do not have prostate glands and anyway cancer cannot be 'caught' from another person.

18.   *My father is due to have radiotherapy for prostate cancer. He has been told he will need treatment sessions every weekday for about six weeks. As it will be difficult for him to get to the hospital each day, is it possible for him to have one large dose of radiotherapy rather than several small ones?*

Normal cells are able to repair themselves to some extent after smaller doses of radiation, whereas malignant cells are not and are gradually killed off. However, one large dose of radiation would damage the normal tissue too. Some hospitals and oncology centres have hostel wards where people who are in good health can stay each night during the week while treatment such as radiotherapy continues. Patients are able to come and go as they like but are provided with meals and a bed at night. Your father should ask at the treatment centre if a bed in a hostel ward is available so that he does not have to travel back and forth each day.

19.   *I have been told that after my prostate operation I will have to 'drink plenty' to help flush out my bladder. What sort of drinks are best, and how much is 'plenty'?*

For the first couple of days after your operation you should try to drink up to 3 litres of clear fluid each day. Once the blood has cleared from your urine and you are able to urinate spontaneously again, which may take anything from 24 hours to several days, you can reduce your daily fluid intake to around 1.5 litres. Most types of drink are suitable, including water, tea, coffee, fruit juice and beer.

Case histories

The case histories which follow are not intended to make any specific point. They have been chosen at random as examples of the experiences of different men and are included simply to illustrate the reality of having a prostate operation for these people. Although, by chance, they all involve men in their fifties, prostate surgery is not uncommon up to the age of 80 or even 90.

CASE 1

Martin is 56. During the last couple of years he has experienced intermittent difficulty passing urine, sometimes needing to go the toilet frequently during the day and having to get up several times in the night. His flow of urine was often slow and occasionally he was unable to pass urine at all for several hours. As his symptoms came and went, it was not until he started working as a part-time taxi driver that he decided to seek medical advice. His doctor, suspecting a urinary infection, prescribed a course of antibiotics, but they had no effect.

One evening, having felt the need to urinate frequently during the day but only producing a dribble of urine each time, Martin's condition suddenly became painful and he phoned his doctor who visited him at home. He was taken by ambulance to hospital where a suprapubic catheter was inserted into his bladder through his lower abdominal wall. The catheter produced instant relief and within two days Martin could urinate spontaneously again and was able to go home. While in hospital, he was told that his prostate was enlarged and that an appointment would be made for him at a urology clinic. A couple of weeks later Martin underwent testing at a flow clinic, and a scan confirmed benign prostate enlargement, for which his consultant advised a transurethral resection.

Martin was admitted to hospital some weeks later where he had a chest X-ray, an electrocardiogram and a blood test. He was given an epidural anaesthetic, and his operation was done that afternoon. He awoke with a drip in his arm and a catheter in his bladder. He dozed for the rest of the day but woke up during the night with pain caused by obstruction of the catheter by a blood clot, which was washed out by a nurse. It was the only pain Martin experienced throughout his time in hospital, and he did not require any painkillers. His drip was taken out during the first post-operative morning, and his catheter two days later on the evening before he left hospital.

CASE 2

Tony is 53. He started to develop minor urinary symptoms over a period of several years, eventually needing to urinate every couple of hours or more during the day and having to get up two or three times in the night, sometimes producing only a dribble. About a year ago, he went to his family doctor, who did a blood test and sent him to hospital for a scan. The results of both tests were clear, ruling out prostate cancer, and Tony decided to put up with his problems.

A couple of months later, he started taking zinc tablets which he bought over the counter in a pharmacy and which, after several weeks, seemed to be improving his symptoms slightly. He continued to take the tablets for a few months until one day, having had to get up to urinate five or six times during the night and producing only a dribble of urine, he developed quite severe pain in his lower abdomen and was unable to pass any urine at all, despite a desperate urge to do so. Tony rang his doctor and made an appointment to see him the following day. However, the situation deteriorated during the afternoon until he was unable to sit down and had a constant ache and periodic spasms of pain. That evening, he went to his doctor who inserted a urinary catheter to relieve his very swollen and tender bladder. A catheter bag was strapped to Tony's lower leg and he was given a larger bag to attach at night. The district nurse visited him at home the following day.

Tony was admitted to a private hospital two days later, and underwent a transurethral resection of his prostate the following morning. He chose to have a general anaesthetic, and came round after the operation feeling quite well but with a tender groin, which was relieved by analgesic tablets. He was also given an antibiotic injection after his operation.

The catheter was removed two days later, which Tony found to be a brief but painful experience. He was then able to urinate spontaneously, passing several small pieces of prostate tissue. The amount of urine he produced increased during the day and its colour gradually cleared. He experienced a slight stinging sensation in his penis when urinating, but otherwise felt reasonably well.

CASE 3

William is 55. He had experienced some degree of difficulty urinating, with a slow rate of flow, for several years. About six months ago, he began to have to get up several times in the night but it was not until he had done so 14 times one night that he decided to consult his family doctor. Suspecting an enlarged prostate, William's doctor referred him to a consultant who recommended a transurethral resection. The operation was done using a spinal anaesthetic. Following surgery, William found it very painful to urinate for some time and had quite severe pains in his lower abdomen for about six weeks but, assuming this was normal, he did not seek advice. His urinary problems were much improved after the operation and he regained complete bladder control.

However, when the pieces of prostate tissue which had been resected were examined, some were found to be cancerous. Further tests were done, including blood tests, a magnetic resonance imaging scan and an isotope bone scan, and no signs of metastases were detected. William's consultant told him that it could be many years before the cancer caused him any problems, if at all, or the situation could change and it could spread. In view of his relatively young age, he was asked to consider the possibility of having a radical prostatectomy. William took several months to make up his mind, but finally decided to opt for surgery.

Some six months after his first operation, he underwent a radical prostatectomy under a general anaesthetic. He was also given an epidural for pain relief which was removed about 48 hours after the operation, at the same time as his drip and wound drain. His pelvic lymph nodes were also removed and examined for any signs of regional spread of the cancer.

When William came round from the anaesthetic, he had very little pain and no sickness. However, once the epidural had been removed, he did suffer pain in his abdomen and continued to take pain-killing tablets for several days.

A couple of days after surgery, William experienced the same severe pain he had had after his transurethral resection which his consultant diagnosed as due to muscular bladder spasms. He was given a suppository which eased the pain almost immediately, and thereafter took pills regularly for several days to prevent it returning.

On the first couple of post-operative days, William felt pretty miserable and uncomfortable. A physiotherapist visited him the day after his operation to get him up and help him take a few steps. She returned the following day when he was able to walk a little more without feeling dizzy, and after that he could shower and walk around his room alone. She visited him daily, to check his breathing and encourage him to do deep breathing exercises, until he left hospital six days after his operation.

William found it difficult to sleep in hospital, but it was not until the night before he went home that he asked for sleeping tablets.

He was told that his catheter would have to remain in place for three weeks, until he had had further tests. He was advised not to drive until it had been removed as he would find it difficult to make an emergency stop without hurting himself.

William had quite severe wind after his operation. He was surprised by the amount of pain he experienced in his abdomen, which he was advised might not clear completely for about a month.

CASE 4

Peter is 50. About five years ago he started to pass urine more frequently than normal, eventually often having to get up two or three times in the night. When his problems began to interfere with his daily life, he went to his family doctor who referred him to a consultant. A manual rectal examination revealed an enlarged prostate, and Peter attended a flow clinic where he had several tests, including a transrectal ultrasound scan. The level of PSA in his blood was high, but a biopsy showed no sign of cancer.

Shortly afterwards, Peter underwent a transurethral resection, but when the tissue removed from his prostate was examined, it confirmed that he did, in fact, have prostate cancer. A couple of months later he had a radical prostatectomy under a general anaesthetic. He had little pain following his operation, although he found the catheter irritating and uncomfortable.

Peter had check-ups every two months for a while (at each of which his PSA level was found to be normal) and will contine to have them once a year for the time being. Some three years after his radical prostatectomy, he feels well and there are no signs that the cancer has spread.

Medical terms

Abscess A collection of pus secondary to localised infection.

Adenocarcinoma A malignant tumour (cancer) of glandular epithelial tissue. It is the most common type of prostate cancer.

Adjuvant therapy A treatment used in combination with another, primary, treatment to enhance its efficacy.

Allergy An abnormal reaction to a substance. An allergic reaction can be mild, causing an itchy rash, or severe, leading to fainting, vomiting, loss of consciousness or, rarely, death.

Alpha blocker A drug which obstructs the passage of impulses between the alpha receptors of nerves. Alpha receptors receive the nerve stimulation to the muscles within the prostate gland. If they are blocked, the muscles (and therefore the prostate itself) relax, reducing the resistance to urine flow.

Anaesthesia The absence of sensation.

Anaesthetic A drug which causes loss of sensation in part or all of the body.

Anaesthetist A doctor trained in the administration of anaesthetics.

Analgesic A drug which blocks the sensation of pain; a painkiller.

Antibiotic A substance which kills bacteria or prevents them multiplying or growing.

Anticholinergic drug A drug which suppresses the action of acetylcholine which is present in the tissues of the body and which transmits nerve impulses at certain sites.

Anticoagulant A substance which prevents the blood from clotting.

Anti-embolism stockings Stockings sometimes worn during an operation and during any period of immobilisation post-operatively. They assist the circulation of blood in the legs and help to prevent blood clots forming. They are also known as thrombo-embolic deterrent stockings, or TEDS.

Anti-emetic   A drug which helps to reduce feelings of sickness.

Bacteraemia   A condition caused by the presence of bacteria in the circulating blood.

Benign   Non-malignant. A benign disease or condition is likely to respond to appropriate treatment. A benign tumour will remain localised at its site of development and will have no harmful effect other than possibly to interfere with the function of adjacent organs as it grows.

Benign prostatic hyperplasia   The condition that causes enlargement of the prostate which occurs in men with increasing age.

Biopsy   The surgical removal of a piece of tissue from a living body for examination under a microscope to assist or confirm a diagnosis.

Bladder neck incision   An operation which involves making a cut in the neck of the bladder or along the prostate gland to improve the symptoms of benign prostatic hyperplasia. It is sometimes the treatment of choice for a prostate gland which is not significantly enlarged.

Cancer   A malignant growth resulting from the uncontrolled multiplication of cells which fail to die naturally. If left untreated, the cancer cells may invade nearby areas of the body and eventually spread to distant sites.

Cannula   A very fine tube or needle. Fluids can be introduced into or removed from the body through an intravenous cannula which has been inserted into a vein, usually in the back of the hand, and anaesthetic drugs are administered through it during an operation. Cannulae are usually made of plastic, but used to be metal or glass.

Carcinoma   A cancer in epithelial tissue, such as that of the prostate gland or bladder. Carcinomas are always malignant, but their severity and tendency to spread can vary.

Catheter   A thin tube used to withdraw or introduce fluid into the body. Urinary catheters are usually inserted into the bladder via the urethra to drain the urine from it. Suprapubic catheters are inserted directly into the bladder through a small hole made in the lower abdominal wall.

Catheterisation   The passing of a catheter.

Cauterise   To burn a part with heat or some other agent. The severed ends of small blood vessels are sealed with the tip of an instrument heated by an electric current to stop them bleeding during surgery.

Chemotherapy   Treatment with drugs, usually anti-cancer drugs.

Clinical nurse specialist   A nurse with specialist knowledge who works closely with doctors and patients in a particular field of medicine and who is able to spend time talking to patients and answering their questions.

Complication   An adverse condition which occurs as the result of another disease or condition. It may also occur after an operation or treatment.

Computer tomography (CT)   A scan which takes X-ray images through 'slices' of the body. The images are interpreted by a computer to build up a three-dimensional picture.

Connective tissue   Fibrous tissue which connects and supports organs within the body.

Consent form   A form which patients must sign before surgery to confirm that they understand what is involved in their operation and give their consent for it to take place. Signing the form also gives consent for the use of anaesthetic drugs and any other procedures which doctors feel to be necessary during surgery.

Constipation   Difficulty or infrequent opening of the bowels or retention of faeces. The condition can sometimes be relieved by a high-fibre diet or laxatives.

Consultant An experienced and fully trained doctor who specialises in a particular type of medicine.

Cystitis Inflammation of the bladder due to injury or infection.

Cystogram A series of X-rays taken following the introduction of a dye into the bladder. The X-rays are taken as the bladder empties and reveal any holes in the urethra through which urine is escaping.

Cystoscope A telescope-like surgical instrument with a light attached which can be inserted through the urethra to examine the bladder. Other instruments can be introduced through it as required.

Deep vein thrombosis (DVT) A blood clot in a deep vein, often in the lower leg or pelvis.

Defaecate To empty the bowels.

Detrusor decompensation Inability of the muscles of the bladder to contract properly which causes the bladder to become floppy and unable to expel urine.

Detrusor instability Overactivity of the muscular layer of the bladder wall which makes the bladder try to empty itself at inappropriate times. It can cause symptoms such as frequency, urgency, nocturia and urge incontinence.

Diagnosis The identification of a disease based on its symptoms and signs.

Diarrhoea The frequent passage of unformed faeces.

Diathermy A method of generating heat by means of a high-frequency electric current. It is used in surgery to destroy diseased tissue or to stop bleeding from damaged blood vessels.

Discharge letter A letter given to patients leaving hospital (or sent directly from the hospital) to deliver to their family doctor. It gives details of treatment and any necessary follow-up.

Distant metastasis Spread of malignant cells via the blood or lymphatic vessels to sites which are distant from the primary cancer.

Diuretic   A substance which increases the volume of urine produced.

Drain   Often a tube, which may be attached to a bag or bottle, which is inserted near a wound to drain away excess blood and fluid.

Drip/Intravenous infusion   A tube through which fluid is administered to replace that lost from the body after an operation or injury. One end is inserted into a vein in the arm and the other end is attached to a bottle or bag containing a specially balanced saline or sugar solution.

Efferent duct   The duct which carries sperm from the seminiferous tubules in the testis to the epididymis.

Ejaculation   The sudden ejection of semen from the penis following sexual arousal.

Ejaculatory duct   The duct which carries semen from the seminal vesicle to the urethra in the penis.

Electrocardiogram (ECG)   The activity of the heart recorded as a series of electrical wave patterns.

Electrocautery   The application of the electrically heated tip of an instrument to the ends of blood vessels to stop them bleeding.

Embolus (plural: **emboli**)   A piece of a blood clot (or air bubble) which has broken away and can pass through the blood vessels. If it lodges in a vital organ, such as the lung, it can have fatal consequences.

Epididymis   A mass of tissue attached to the border of the testis which is composed of tightly coiled efferent ducts carrying sperm which have been produced in the testis.

Epidural anaesthetic   An anaesthetic drug which is injected into the space around the nerves in the back. It causes numbness in the legs and groin which lasts for three to five hours. Epidurals are used for pain relief and/or to produce loss of sensation during surgery to the legs or lower body.

Excision   Removal by cutting.

Fertility   In men – the capacity to induce conception; in women – the capacity to conceive and give birth. A man's fertility is dependent on the number and quality of his sperm and not on his ability to perform the sexual act.

Fixed Price Care   The system used by some private hospitals whereby a fixed price is quoted for a particular type of operation and some of the hospitalisation costs associated with it.

Flow clinic   A urology clinic at which various tests are done to investigate the cause of urinary symptoms.

Frequency (of micturition)   The number of times the bladder needs to be emptied. Increased frequency can occur with various urinary and prostate conditions.

General anaesthetic   A drug which induces loss of consciousness and abolishes the sensation of pain in all parts of the body.

Gonorrhoea   An inflammatory disease of the genito-urinary tract caused by a micro-organism which is usually transmitted during sexual intercourse. A type of venereal disease.

Haematoma   A blood-filled swelling. A haematoma can form after trauma or in a wound after an operation if blood continues to leak from a blood vessel. If the blood spreads in the tissues, it appears as a bruise.

Heparin   A substance which occurs naturally in the body and which helps to prevent the blood clotting. It may be given in low doses by injection before and after surgery to people who are at particular risk of developing blood clots, for example during long periods of immobilisation. Higher doses of heparin are given once a blood clot has formed to try to prevent it getting worse.

Hesitancy (of micturition)   Difficulty in passing urine which may result in a slow rate of flow.

Histological examination   The microscopic examination of a sample of tissue which has been taken from the body by biopsy.

Hormone therapy   Treatment with drugs which affect the hormones which regulate the growth and function of organs. For example, drugs can be given to relieve the symptoms caused by a prostate cancer by suppressing the production of the hormone testosterone by the testes and thus slowing the rate of growth of the cancer.

Hospice   A centre which provides medical care and various non-medical facilities for those with terminal illness and their families. Hospice staff help people to lead full and independent lives for as long as possible by giving them wide-ranging support, in some cases for many years.

Hostel ward   A hospital ward set aside for people who do not need medical care but who are unable to go home immediately after an operation or between treatment sessions. Food and a bed are provided, but although there is always someone in charge of the ward it does not have a full medical staff.

Hydronephrosis   Dilatation of the drainage system of the kidneys which is caused by the accumulation of fluid and leads to enlargement of the kidneys themselves.

Hypertrophy   Enlargement of an organ caused by an increase in the number and size of its cells.

Immunological treatment/Immunotherapy   Treatment (usually involving the use of drugs) which activates the body's own immune mechanisms to fight disease.

Impotence   Inability to get an erection. It is sometimes a side-effect of prostate surgery.

Incision   A cut or wound made by a sharp instrument, such as during an operation.

Incontinence   The lack of voluntary control over the discharge of urine or faeces.

Induction agent   A drug used in anaesthesia to bring on loss of consciousness.

Inguinal canal   A canal which runs from the abdomen, through the groin and into the scrotum and through which the testis descends in a male fetus before birth.

Inhalational anaesthetic   An anaesthetic given as a mixture of gases which is inhaled, usually to maintain anaesthesia.

Intra-operative   Occurring during an operation.

Intravenous anaesthetic   A general anaesthetic drug which is injected into a vein via a cannula, usually in the back of the hand.

Intravenous pyelogram (IVP)   An X-ray taken following the injection of a special dye into a vein in the arm which enters the kidneys and is excreted via the ureters into the bladder.

Irritable bladder   Overactivity of the muscles of the wall of the bladder causing it to try to empty at inappropriate times.

Keyhole surgery   A colloquial name for laparoscopic surgery.

Laparoscopic surgery   Surgery done with the aid of a tele-scope-like instrument called a **laparoscope.** The laparoscope has a light source and a camera attached and is introduced through a small hole in the body wall to enable the surgeon to examine the internal organs. Surgical instruments are inserted through similar small incisions. Because there is no large wound post-operatively, recovery time is reduced.

Laser treatment   The destruction of tissue using lasers. The laser contains substances which, when stimulated by light energy, emit a beam of light of great intensity which can be directed precisely. Laser treatment can be used to destroy tissue from an enlarged prostate without causing bleeding.

Leakage of urine   The dribbling of urine before or after urinating.

Lesion   Any abnormality such as an injury, infection or tumour.

Libido   Sexual desire.

Local anaesthetic   An anaesthetic which numbs the area of the body around which it is injected.

Local injection   An injection of a substance which remains confined to one area and is not distributed throughout the body.

Local metastasis   Spread of malignant cells which is confined to the area immediately around the primary site.

Lymph   A pale-coloured fluid which flows within the lymphatic vessels of the body and is eventually returned to the blood. It contains disease-fighting cells, the lymphocytes.

Lymph node A gland through which lymph flows and is filtered and which acts as a repository for the lymphocytes.

Lymphadenectomy Surgical removal of lymph nodes for examination when regional spread of cancer is suspected.

Lymphangiogram A test done to detect spread of cancer to the lymph nodes. A special dye is injected into the lymphatic system which highlights the lymph vessels and nodes on X-ray.

Lymphocyte A type of white blood cell involved in fighting disease in the body.

Magnetic resonance imaging (MRI) The use of a large magnet to produce a magnetic field in individual cells of the body. An energy field is applied which affects the alignment of atoms within the cells and causes them to emit a signal which is detected and interpreted as an image of the body.

Maintenance agent A drug used during an operation to maintain the state of general anaesthesia.

Malignant Used to describe a lesion which is likely to spread locally and to distant parts of the body – a cancer.

Metastasis (noun) (plural: **metastases**) A secondary cancer at a site distant from the original (primary) cancer.

Metastasis (verb) The spread of cancerous cells through the blood or lymphatic vessels from the site of the original cancer.

Metastasise To spread to a distant part.

Metastatic disease Advanced cancer due to the spread of malignant cells from the primary lesion.

Microwave treatment The use of microwave radiation to destroy tissue selectively without causing bleeding. The treatment is sometimes used to remove tissue from an enlarged prostate gland, the instrument delivering the microwaves being inserted through the rectum or urethra.

Micturition The act of passing urine; urination.

Nasogastric tube A tube inserted via a nostril after some operations to drain the stomach and prevent vomiting. A smaller version is sometimes used to provide a specially balanced fluid to patients who are unable to eat.

National Health Service (NHS) The system of medical care, set up in Britain in 1948, under which medical treatment is mostly funded by taxation.

Nausea A feeling of sickness.

Neuroma A tumour of nerve cells and nerve fibres.

Nil by mouth A term used to mean that no food or drink should be swallowed in the hours before an operation.

Nocturia Having to get up at night to pass urine (often small amounts) due to an irritation of the bladder or a prostate problem.

Nocturnal polyuria The passage of large amounts of urine at night because the kidneys are producing more than they normally would at night.

Obesity An excessive amount of fat in the body. This term is non-specific and is being replaced by a figure calculated from height and weight measurements, known as the **body mass index**.

Oncologist A physician specialising in the treatment of tumours, particularly cancer.

Oncology The study and management of new growths; the study of cancer.

Open prostatectomy Surgery to remove tissue from a very large prostate gland which is done through an incision made in the abdominal wall.

Orchidectomy Surgical removal of a testis. **Bilateral orchidectomy** (removal of both testes) is a type of hormone therapy sometimes undertaken to treat prostate cancer by reducing the level of testosterone on which the cancer depends.

Palliative therapy Treatment used to alleviate symptoms but which cannot cure the condition which causes them.

Penis The male sexual organ which becomes enlarged and

erect as a result of sexual arousal and through which semen is ejected. The urethra, via which urine also leaves the body, runs through the penis in men.

Perineum   The area of the body between the scrotum and anus.

Post-operative   Following an operation.

Pre-clerking admission procedure   A procedure used in some hospitals whereby patients attend an appointment a few days before an operation for pre-operative tests, such as blood tests and ECGs, the results of which are thus available when the patient is admitted for surgery.

Pre-medication ('Pre-med.')   A drug which is given before another drug, for example one given an hour or two before an operation to relax the patient before anaesthesia is started.

Pre-operative   Before an operation.

Primary tumour   The first (and sometimes only) or most important tumour to develop.

Prognosis   An opinion about the probable course and final outcome of a disease which is made when all the known facts are considered.

Prophylaxis   Preventative treatment.

Prostate gland   The gland which surrounds the neck of the bladder and urethra in men and secretes a fluid which forms part of the semen. It often enlarges in elderly men, causing constriction of the urethra and thus urinary symptoms.

Prostate specific antigen (PSA)   A component in the blood of men which increases with various prostate diseases. It may be significantly raised with prostate cancer.

Prostatectomy   Surgical removal of part or all of the prostate gland.

Prostatic acid phosphatase (PAP)   A component of the blood of men which may increase in association with advanced prostate cancer.

Prostatism   A syndrome caused by enlargement of the prostate gland which leads to urinary obstruction, and thus to retention of urine, hesitancy, urgency and nocturia.

Prostatitis Inflammation of the prostate gland which may or may not be due to bacterial infection but which can be treated with antibiotics. Its symptoms are similar to those of prostate enlargement.

Prostatotomy An operation done to relieve the symptoms caused by a slightly enlarged prostate. It involves making one or two cuts along the length of the prostate gland so that it falls away from the urethra, allowing urine to flow unobstructed.

Pulmonary embolism A blood clot or air bubble which blocks the blood vessels in the lung.

Pyrexia A fever.

Radiation oncologist A radiotherapist.

Radical prostatectomy Surgical removal of the entire prostate gland, its capsule and the seminal vesicles. It involves making a long, vertical incision in the abdomen and is sometimes used to treat prostate cancer in its early stages of development.

Radical treatment Aggressive treatment aimed at curing a serious illness.

Radiographer A technician qualified to make X-ray examinations.

Radiologist A doctor trained in the use of X-radiation for diagnostic purposes.

Radiotherapist/Radiation oncologist A doctor specialising in the use of radiation as treatment, for example for cancer.

Radiotherapy Treatment with radiation.

Recovery room A ward near the operating theatre to which patients are taken after surgery so that they can be watched closely while they recover from a general anaesthetic.

Rectal examination The insertion of a finger through the rectum to feel the prostate.

Recurrence The reappearance of symptoms or signs of a disease after a period of apparent recovery.

Regional metastasis   Spread of malignant cells to nearby sites, usually the nearest lymph nodes.

Regression   The disappearance or reduction of the symptoms and signs of a disease.

Resectoscope   A surgical instrument inserted through the urethra to cut away (resect) part of the prostate during transurethral resection.

Retention (of urine)   The holding back of urine in the bladder due to obstruction or muscular weakness of the bladder wall. Acute retention can have serious consequences but can be relieved by the passage of a catheter, either through the urethra or suprapubically, to empty the bladder.

Retrograde ejaculation   The passage of sperm back up the urethra into the bladder during ejaculation. It is sometimes a side-effect of prostate surgery and causes reduced fertility.

Scrotum   A pouch of skin present in men which is divided into two by a septum, each half containing a testis, epididymis and the lower part of the spermatic cord.

Secondary tumour   A tumour at a site distant from that of the original (primary) tumour; a metastasis.

Semen   The fluid containing sperm and secretions from the prostate and seminal vesicles.

Seminal vesicle   A coiled tube at the base of the bladder, adjacent to the prostate, which stores semen.

Seminiferous tubule   A tube in the testis in which sperm are produced. Each testis contains one to three of these tightly coiled tubules.

Septicaemia   Severe infection caused by large numbers of bacteria in the blood which multiply and spread.

Seroma   A collection of clear fluid, such as lymph, which may develop following an operation. If persistent, the fluid can be drawn off with a needle.

Side-effect   An effect other than that desired which results from the use of a drug or other form of treatment.

Sign   Something a doctor looks for as an indication of disease, such as a lesion or swelling.

Sperm   The mature male cell which contains male genetic material capable of developing into a new individual when united with a female egg. It consists of a small head region, a short middle piece, and a mobile tail which enables it to swim.

Spermatic cord   The cord containing the nerves, blood and lymphatic vessels supplying the testis.

Spinal anaesthetic   An anaesthetic which is injected between the vertebrae of the spine into the space around the nerves in the back. It causes numbness in the legs and groin which lasts for three to five hours.

Staging   Classification of the development of a disease, i.e. whether it is localised, has spread regionally or to distant sites in the body. The stage at which a cancer is first detected may have a bearing on the likely outcome of its treatment.

Stent   A small coil or spiral which can be inserted into the top of the urethra to keep the sphincter into the bladder open and thus relieve obstruction. The use of stents is less effective than surgery and tends to be reserved for older men with urinary symptoms whose general health is poor.

Steroid   One of a group of naturally occurring substances in the body which includes the sex hormones.

Suture   A surgical stitch or row of stitches.

Symptom   Something experienced by a patient which indicates a disturbance of normal body function, for example pain or nausea.

Testis   The male reproductive organ in which sperm develop; the testicle.

Testosterone   The male sex hormone (a steroid) produced by the testes, which, amongst other things, plays a role in regulating the growth and function of the prostate.

Thrombo-embolic deterrent stockings (TEDS)   See Anti-embolism stockings.

Thrombosis   The coagulation of blood within a vein or artery which produces a blood clot.

Thrombus   A blood clot which forms in, and remains in, a blood vessel or the heart.

Topical anaesthetic   An anaesthetic which remains localised in the area it is applied.

Transrectal ultrasonography   An ultrasound scan of the lower abdomen for which the scanning device is inserted into the rectum.

Transurethral resection of the prostate (TURP)   The surgical removal of part of the prostate gland. The surgical instruments are introduced via the urethra and therefore the operation does not involve incision of the abdominal wall. Insertion of a small telescope allows the surgeon to view the organs and the operation as it progresses on a video or television monitor in the operating theatre.

Tumour   A swelling; an abnormal growth of cells which can be benign or malignant. A **benign tumour** remains localised and does not spread to other parts of the body. It has no harmful effect except possibly to compress adjacent organs as it enlarges. A **malignant tumour** (a cancer) will invade the surrounding tissues, interfering with their normal functioning. Cells from it may also spread to other parts of the body, giving rise to secondary tumours.

Ultrasonography   *See* Ultrasound scan.

Ultrasound scan/Ultrasonography   The passage of high-frequency sound waves through the body wall which are reflected back from solid objects and enable an image of the internal organs to be built up by a computer.

Ureter   The duct which transports urine from the kidney to the bladder.

Urethra   The canal which carries urine from the bladder to the exterior. In men it also transports semen during ejaculation.

Urge incontinence   The leakage of urine following a sudden need to urinate.

Urgency (of micturition) Difficulty controlling the sudden (and possibly frequent) need to pass urine.

Urinary incompetence Failure of the sphincter at the base of the bladder to close, leading to urinary incontinence of some degree.

Urinary obstruction Obstruction of the bladder which prevents the free passage of urine through the urethra.

Urinary stasis The retention of a volume of urine in the bladder following urination.

Urine flow test Measurement of the volume and rate of flow of urine as it is passed into a funnel-shaped container attached to a meter.

Urodynamics Special tests to measure the pressures in the bladder and prostate gland to discover the cause of urinary symptoms. The tests are often done for people with incontinence, and sometimes if obstruction by the prostate is suspected by not confirmed by other means. A tiny catheter is passed into the bladder which is filled up. The pressures are measured while the bladder is filling and again when urine is passed. The tests may be combined with **video urodynamics** for which a dye is put into the bladder which is viewed on a video screen as it empties.

Urologist A doctor with specific training in, and experience of, problems of the urinary system.

Vas deferens (plural: **vasa deferentia**) The tube which carries sperm from the testis to the penis.

Watchful waiting The regular monitoring of a condition causing mild to moderate symptoms. It may be appropriate for an older man with a small, slow-growing prostate cancer or for someone who is unfit for surgery.

X-ray A type of electromagnetic radiation of short wavelength which is able to pass through opaque bodies. It can be used in diagnosis, by allowing the visualisation of internal structures and organs of the body, or in higher doses as therapy to destroy malignant cells.

Useful addresses

The organisations listed here are good starting points for those wanting further information, advice and support. Only a few have been set up to help people with specific prostate-related or incontinence problems, and these addresses are given at the beginning of the list for each country. Inevitably, men with prostate cancer and their families are most likely to seek advice and support, and the majority of the addresses are therefore for the more general cancer organisations.

BRITAIN

Incontinence Information Helpline: 0191 2130050
Services available: a confidential helpline for people with bladder and bowel problems. Open weekdays from 2 to 7 p.m.

The Continence Foundation
2 Doughty Street
London WC1N 2PH
Helpline: 0191 2130050
Services available: confidential advice for people with bladder and bowel problems.

The Association of Continence Advisers
c/o Disabled Living Foundation
380-384 Harrow Road
London W9 2HU
Telephone: 0171 2896111

Services available: a list of continence advisers and a directory of continence aids.

Newcastle Council for the Disabled
Continence Advisory Service
The Dene Centre
Castles Farm Road
Newcastle upon Tyne NE3 1PH
Services available: advice about the financial benefits and services available for people with incontinence.

Institute of Psychosexual Medicine
11 Chandos Street
London W1M 9DE
Telephone: 0171 580 0631
Services available: lists of doctors trained in psychosexual medicine. Write to request names of doctors in your area.

The Prostate Cancer Charity
Ducane Road
London W12 0NN
Telephone: 0181 259 8124
Services available: information about prostate cancer. Write for details enclosing a first-class stamp.

The British Association of Cancer United Patients (BACUP)
3 Bath Place
Rivington Street
London EC2A 3JR
Telephone: 0171 613 2121
Freephone for patients, counselling service: 0800 181199
Services available: cancer information; booklets; details of cancer help organisations in different areas. Enquiries made

by telephone or letter are answered by experienced cancer nurses.

Cancerlink
17 Britannia Street
London WC1X 9JN
Phone: 0171 833 2451
Services available: emotional support, advice and information about all aspects of cancer; a range of free booklets on cancer; help to anyone wanting to set up a cancer support group.

Cancer Relief Macmillan Fund
Anchor House
15/19 Britten Street
London SW3 3TZ
Telephone: 0171 351 7811
Services available: a variety of services for people with cancer and their families; information about Macmillan nurses and the care they can offer.

Hospice Information Service
St Christopher's Hospice
51-59 Lawrie Park Road
Sydenham
London SE26 6DZ
Telephone: 0181 778 9252
Services available: a directory with details of hospices, home care teams and hospital support teams; information on local services.

Institute for Complementary Medicine
PO Box 194
London SE16 1Q2
Services available: a list of reliable practitioners of various kinds of

complementary medicine; details of support groups. Requests for information should be sent in writing, enclosing a stamped, addressed envelope.

Irish Cancer Society
Information Officer
5 Northumberland Road
Dublin 4
Telephone: 1 681855
Helpline: 1 681233
Services available: a helpline service staffed by nurses who can give information on all aspects of cancer and details of support groups; night-time nursing care for people in their own homes which must be requested by a doctor or public health nurse.

The Ulster Cancer Foundation
40–42 Eglantine Avenue
Belfast BT9 6DX
Telephone: 01232 663281/2/3
Helpline: 01232 663449
Services available: an information helpline, open every weekday morning, staffed by experienced cancer nurses; counselling at the centre.

Tak Tent Cancer Support Organisation
G Block
Western Infirmary
Glasgow G11 6NT
Telephone: 0141 334 6699 or 0141 357 4519
Services available: emotional support, counselling and information on cancer and its treatment; courses for cancer sufferers and their families; details of support groups throughout Scotland.

Tenovus Cancer Information Centre
142 Whitchurch Road
Cardiff CF4 3NA
Telephone: 01222 619846
Helpline: 01222 691998
Services available: information, support and counselling provided by cancer sufferers and their families; a drop-in centre and a helpline staffed by a trained cancer nurse.

AUSTRALIA

Australian Cancer Society
Angus & Coote Building
500 George Street
Sydney
New South Wales 2000
Telephone: 02 267 1944

Anti-Cancer Council of Victoria
1 Rathdowne Street
Carlton
South Victoria 3053
Telephone: 03 662 3300

Anti-Cancer Foundation of the Universities of South Australia
24 Brougham Place
North Adelaide
South Australia 5006
Telephone: 08 267 5222

Cancer Foundation of Western Australia Inc.
42 Ord Street
West Perth

Western Australia 6005
Telephone: 09 321 6224

Northern Territory Anti-Cancer Foundation
Shop 24
Casuarina Plaza
Casuarina
Northern Territory 0810
Telephone: 08 927 4888

Queensland Cancer Fund
553 Gregory Terrace
Fortitude Valley
Queensland 4006
Telephone: 07 257 1155

Tasmanian Cancer Committee
43 Collins Street
Hobart
Tasmania 7000
Telephone: 002 30 0895

NEW ZEALAND

Cancer Society of New Zealand Inc.
Molesworthy House
101-105 Molesworthy Street
P.O. Box 12145
Wellington
New Zealand
Telephone: 4 4736409

CANADA

International Prostate Centre
71 King Street West
Suite 504
Mississauga
Ontario L5B 4A2
Telephone: 905 275 8868

Toronto Hospital Prostate Clinic
200 Elizabeth Street
Toronto
Ontario M5G 2C4
Telephone: 416 340 4800, Ext. 3644

Mississauga Prostate Cancer Group
c/o Canadian Cancer Society
1140 Burnamthorpe Road West
Suite 106
Mississauga
Ontario L5C 4EP
Telephone: 905 896 3200

The **Canadian Cancer Society** is a national organization. It provides a range of services for people living with cancer, their families and friends. It has more than 3000 contact points around the country, and the following offices.

Chimo Building, 2nd Floor
P.O. Box 8921
Freshwater & Crosbie Road
St John's
Newfoundland A1B 3R9
Telephone: 709 753 6520

1 Rochford Street, Suite #1
Charlottetown
Prince Edward Island C1A 3T1
Telephone: 902 566 4007

5826 South Street, Suite 1
Halifax
Nova Scotia B3H 1S6
Telephone: 902 423 6183

133 Prince William Street
P.O. Box 2089
Saint John
New Brunswick E2L 3T6
Telephone: 506 634 6272

Maison de la societe canadienne du cancer
5151 Boul. l'Assumption
Montreal
Quebec H1T 4A9
Telephone: 514 255 5151

1639 Yonge Street
Toronto
Ontario M4T 2W6
Telephone: 416 488 5400

193 Sherbrook Street
Winnipeg
Manitoba R3C 2B7
Telephone: 204 774 7483

2445 13th Avenue, Suite 201
Regina
Saskatchewan S4P 0W1
Telephone: 306 757 4260

#200, 2424 4th Street S.W.
Calgary
Alberta T2S 2T4
Telephone: 403 228 4487

565 West Tenth Avenue
Vancouver
British Columbia V5Z 4J4
Telephone: 604 872 4400

NORTH AMERICA

The following are just a few examples of the many organizations in the USA. Your local **State Department of Health** should be able to supply further addresses of appropriate centers in your area.

American Foundation for Urologic Disease
300 W. Pratt Street
Suite 401
Baltimore
Maryland 21201
Telephone (toll free): 800 242 2383

American Prostate Society
1340 Charwood Road
Suite F
Hanover
Maryland 21076
Telephone (toll free): 800 678 1238

Continence Restored Inc.
785 Park Avenue
New York
New York 10021
Telephone: 212 879 3131

Help for Incontinent People
PO Box 544
Union
SC 29379
Telephone: 803 579 7900

International Health Council
P.O. Box 151
Fairbanks
Alaska 99707

National Kidney and Urologic Diseases Information Clearing House
9000 Rockville Pike
Box NKUDIC
Bethesda
Maryland 20892
Telephone: 301 654 4415

Simon Foundation for Continence
Box 815
Wilmette
Illinois 60091
Telephone: 708 864 3913

American Cancer Society
1599 Clifton Road NE
Atlanta
Georgia 30329
Telephone: 404 320 3333

Cancer Care
1180 Avenue of the Americas
New York
New York 10036
Telephone: 212 221 3300

Cancer Control Society
2043 N. Berendo Street
Los Angeles
California 90027
Telephone: 213 663 7801

Cancer Information Service
Office of Cancer Communication
NCI/NIH, Building 31, 10A07
9000 Rockville Pike
Bethesda
Maryland 20892

R.A. Bloch Cancer Foundation
4410 Main
Kansas City
Missouri 64111
Telephone: 816 932 8453

How to complain

If you are unhappy about anything that has occurred – or, indeed, that has not occurred – during your stay in hospital, there are several possible paths to follow if you want to make a complaint.

However, before you set the complaints machinery in motion, you should give careful thought to what is involved. Once a formal complaint has been made against a doctor and the complaints procedure has begun, there is little chance of stopping it.

If you think you have a genuine grievance, do try to talk to the person concerned, explaining as clearly and unemotionally as possible what it is that you feel has gone wrong. If you do not feel able to discuss things directly, you can always present your case in a letter.

The vast majority of doctors – family doctors and those who work in hospitals – are dedicated, conscientious and hard working. They really do have their patients' best interests at heart, and many work very long hours each week, night and day. A complaint against a doctor is usually a devastating blow, which can cause considerable stress. Of course, if something has gone wrong during your medical treatment, you may also have suffered stress and unhappiness, but before you make an official complaint, do consider whether your doctor's actions have really warranted what many would see as a 'kick in the teeth'.

The best approach is to make a polite and reasoned enquiry to the person concerned. However angry or irritated you may feel, a complaint made aggressively, however justified this may seem, is unlikely to achieve much.

The following brief sections explain how to make an official complaint in the UK. Leaflets and other information giving details of all the appropriate councils and complaints procedures and how they work can be obtained from your hospital or local health authority. If you have any problems with the offices mentioned below, information about what to do and who to go to for help is available from Citizens' Advice Bureaus and Community Health Councils.

HOSPITAL STAFF

If your complaint concerns something that has happened during your stay in hospital and for some reason you are unable to approach the person directly concerned, you can talk to the ward sister or charge nurse, the hospital doctor on your ward, or the senior manager for the department or ward. Many complaints can be dealt with directly by one of these people, but if this is not possible, they will be able to refer you to the appropriate person.

THE GENERAL MANAGER

If you are intimidated by the thought of speaking to one of the people mentioned above, you can write to the hospital's General Manager, sometimes called the Director of Operations or Chief Executive. The General Manager has responsibility for the way the hospital is run.

The Government's Patients' Charter states that anyone making a complaint about an NHS service must receive a 'full and prompt written reply from the Chief Executive or General Manager'. You should therefore receive an immediate response to your letter, and your complaint should be fully investigated by a senior manager.

The hospital switchboard, or any medical or clerical staff at the hospital, should be able to give you the General Manager's name and office address. If you would prefer to do so, you can make an appointment to speak to him or her, rather than writing a letter.

Depending on how serious your complaint is, you should receive either a full report of the investigation into it or regular letters telling you what is happening until such a report can be made. Do make sure you keep copies of all letters you write and receive concerning your complaint.

DISTRICT HEALTH AUTHORITY

If the treatment you require is not available in your area, or the waiting list is very long, you can contact your local District Health Authority. The District Health Authority is able to deal with complaints concerning the provision of services, rather than with those resulting from something going wrong with your treatment. The District Health Authority can sometimes arrange for you to have treatment elsewhere where waiting lists are shorter, if this is what you want.

Your NHS authority should produce a leaflet to explain how it deals with complaints. This will be available at your hospital or clinic. If you have any difficulty finding out who to contact, write to the General Manager of the hospital. Someone at the hospital will be able to tell you which health authority covers the area in which you live.

COMMUNITY HEALTH COUNCIL

If you would like independent advice and assistance, you can obtain it from your local Community Health Council. Someone from the Community Health Council will be able to explain the complaints procedures to you, help you to write letters to the hospital, and also come with you to any meetings arranged between hospital representatives and yourself. Again, the address of the Community Health Council for your area can be obtained from a hospital or local telephone directory.

REGIONAL MEDICAL OFFICER

If your complaint concerns the standard of *clinical* treatment you received in hospital, and the paths you have already taken have not led to a satisfactory conclusion, you can take it to the Regional Medical Officer for your area.

FAMILY HEALTH SERVICES AUTHORITY

Family doctors are now encouraged to have their own 'in-house' complaints services, but a complaint about your family doctor which you have been unable to sort out by this means can be reported to the Family Health Services Authority. Such complaints should be made within 13 weeks of the incident occurring. Again, your local Community Health Council will be able to give you advice and help you make your complaint and write letters etc.

HEALTH SERVICE COMMISSIONER

If all else has failed, you can take your complaint to the Health Service Commissioner. The commissioner is independent of both the NHS and the government, being responsible to Parliament.

The Health Service Commissioner is able to deal with complaints made by individuals about the failure of a NHS authority to provide the service it should – a failure which has caused actual hardship or injustice. You must have taken your complaint up with your local health authority first, but if you have not received a satisfactory response within a reasonable time, write to the Health Service Commissioner enclosing copies of *all* the relevant letters and documents as well as giving details of the incident itself. The Health Commissioner is not able to investigate complaints about clinical treatment.

You must contact the Health Service Commissioner within *one year* of the incident occurring, unless there is some valid reason why you have been unable to do so.

There is a separate Health Service Commissioner for each country within the United Kingdom.

Health Service Commissioner for England
Church House
Great Smith Street
London SW1P 3BW
Telephone: 0171 276 2035

Health Service Commissioner for Scotland
Second Floor
11 Melville Crescent
Edinburgh EH3 7LU
Telephone: 0131 225 7465

Health Service Commissioner for Wales
4th Floor
Pearl Assurance House
Greyfriars Road
Cardiff CF1 3AG
Telephone: 01222 394621

Office of the Northern Ireland Commissioner for Complaints
33 Wellington Place
Belfast BT1 6HN
Telephone: 01232 233821

TAKING LEGAL ACTION

The legal path is likely to be an expensive one, and should be a last resort rather than a starting point.

In theory, everyone has a right to take legal action. However, unless you have very little money and are entitled to Legal Aid, or a great deal of money, you are unlikely to be able to afford this costly process. The outcome of legal action can never be assured, and the possible cost if you lose your case should be borne in mind.

If you do think you have grounds for compensation for injury caused to you as a result of negligence, advice can be sought from:

The Association for the Victims of Medical Accidents (AVMA)
1 London Road
Forest Hill
London SE23 3TP
Telephone: 0181 291 2793.

Someone from the AVMA will be able to give you free and confidential legal advice about whether or not you have a case worth pursuing. They will also be able to recommend solicitors with training in medical law who may be prepared to represent you.

SUMMARY

Do tell nursing or other medical staff if you are not happy about *any* aspect of your care in hospital. They may be able to deal with your complaint immediately. But do remember, if the matter is a serious one, or if you are not satisfied with the response you receive, you are entitled to pursue it through all the levels that exist to deal with such problems.

Index